THE 15-MINUTE-A-DAY NATURAL FACE LIFT

THE 15-MINUTE-A-DAY NATURAL FACE LIFT

M. J. Saffon

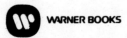 WARNER BOOKS

A Warner Communications Company

*To the lady who encouraged me all the way,
my mother, Mary Saffon,
and the one who is always with me.*

Warner Books Edition

Text copyright © 1979 by M. J. Saffon.
Photographs copyright © 1981 by Warner Books, Inc.

This Warner Books Edition is published by arrangement with
Prentice-Hall, Inc.

Warner Books, Inc., 75 Rockefeller Plaza, New York, N. Y. 10019

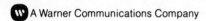 A Warner Communications Company

Printed in the United States of America

First printing: March 1981

10 9 8 7 6 5 4 3 2 1

Book design by Helen Roberts

Cover design by Gene Light

Cover photos by Bill Cadge

Library of Congress Cataloging in Publication Data

Saffon, M J
    The 15-minute-a-day natural face lift.

    Reprint of the ed. published by Prentice-Hall,
Englewood Cliffs, N. J.
    Includes index.
    1. Beauty, Personal.   2. Face — Care and
hygiene.   3. Skin -- Care and hygiene.   4. Exercise.
I. Title.
[RA778.S19   1981]   646.7'26   80-21171
ISBN 0-446-97788-8 (U.S.A.)
ISBN 0-446-97849-3 (Canada)

Acknowledgment

To the great Kathryn Murray,
Emmet B. Groselose, Elizabeth Gilfillan;
they were the greats in facial exercises.
And to all of my wonderful students;
and Julie and Connie who helped me
with the book.

Contents

Beauty, Health, and Your Doctor

I've personally used all of the techniques described in this book, and they have been used successfully by thousands of my clients, students, and even physicians. But everyone is unique, and you should discuss any treatment with your own personal physician.

If you feel dizzy at times, or if your skin itches or has any adverse reaction to any of the methods discussed, discontinue any activity and call your doctor immediately.

This book tells what I do and what works for me and my students; please use caution and good sense in following any directions.

Preface

I'm writing this book because I like people. One of the most satisfying experiences in my life has been seeing my clients, students, and friends grow beautiful and happy, in a very short period of time, through a program of "face building." What could be more rewarding than seeing years slip away and a firm, smooth contour replace a wrinkled brow or sunken cheek?

Before me, my father was also active in the health, beauty, and medical fields. Over the years we've listened to a myriad of problems and been asked thousands of questions. This book comes from those years of experience. My work as a consultant for professional makeup and beauty experts, as well as for thousands of others, has convinced me that anyone and everyone can look, feel, and be more attractive — *almost immediately!*

The 15-minute program was developed for you as a person who is busy and cannot spend the time or money needed to travel to a large city and consult with an expensive expert; so I've tried to design a regimen that can be followed easily, and without your buying equipment or special preparations. You can do everything in your own home.

Another feature of the program is privacy! This program is yours — no one, not even your husband, need know why you suddenly look glowing and smooth, why your hair is shining and your eyes look larger and more lustrous, your brow smoother, your chin firmer.

People often ask when a skin beauty routine should start. At what age does one worry about her looks? Beauty has no age. Young teenagers are often painfully aware of beauty problems. Whether a bridesmaid at an older sister's wedding, or a proud grandmother, we all desire to be attractive.

This book is devoted to firming and filling and beautifying

your facial contours, no matter what your age or sex or skin condition. It uses a combination of massage — the manipulations of the muscles and skin — and exercise — the development of the muscles and skin. You are about to start a carefully planned program of natural face-lifting and facial contour perfection and rejuvenation. The program is planned just for *you*, because you are able to select the massages and exercises that are most suitable for solving your own beauty problems, and you are able to complete the program in the privacy of your own home, in a very short time, using just your own hands.

M. J. Saffon

PART ONE

Before You Begin

Why Does the Skin Age?

Some parts of the body don't seem to age at the same rate as other parts. Certain areas of our bodies remain smooth and firm textured even into old age. The parts of the body that often show age first are the face, neck, and hands.

In order to understand why the face, hands, and neck seem to age the fastest, it is helpful to understand the cause of aging skin. Why lines, wrinkles, sags, pouches, and loss of texture and tone? The reasons for this are many and varied, but there are five main culprits.

First is the weather: nearly all parts of the body are protected by clothing except for the face, neck, and hands. People who work indoors, such as office and factory workers, avoid the worst punishment of the scorching sun and the withering blasts of wind which dry and toughen the skin. Indoor workers generally do not seem to age as fast as farmers, sailors, athletes, or those who are outdoors in every kind of weather over a long period of time.

Second is the lack of muscle tone of the facial and neck muscles: when the facial muscles are not exercised, the muscle fibers deteriorate and shrink, and the skin covering the muscles seems to age very rapidly.

What makes the difference between a young face and an old face? It is the difference in muscle tone and the circulation of the blood through the facial muscles and skin. As the years pass, the supply of blood through the small threadlike capillaries that go to the facial muscles and skin slows. Less oxygen, fewer nutrients, and a diminished supply of blood pass through the muscles and the skin.

Third is gravity: the downward pull that keeps us on earth is an aging factor. This constant pull downward over the years eventually drags the skin downward. The skin sags and there seems to be a lack of firmness and taut smoothness; the face looks old.

Fourth is thirst: without your realizing it, your skin may hunger for water, minerals and other food nutrients, oils, and oxygen. It is through your blood supply that your skin is brought both food nutrients and water. But as you grow older, or if you live in a dry climate, water in lavish and constant supply is needed to keep your skin lustrous and glowing. The skin can be firm and bouncy, that is, elastic, only when its cells contain enough water. Moisture is needed for a youthful skin.

The fifth is you: the way you live, what you eat, your habits can have a dramatic effect on the aging of your skin. Only you can control the gestures and habits that are the cause of aging. Frowning and raising your eyebrows are just bad habits, unnecessary and curable. These actions are careless, senseless contractions that form lines in the forehead prematurely.

Some people call these lines "expression lines." A more descriptive phrase would be "grimaces." The forehead can best convey two expressions: an angry expression, and a look of surprise that is indicated by a lifted eyebrow. Why should you look angry? It only makes you appear unattractive. And, since you are an adult and reasonably sophisticated, why should you be surprised at anything?

Some people grimace and frown repeatedly while they are talking, reading, or watching TV; they are not even aware of it. Probably most facial contortions are performed while talking. The grimace usually comes to emphasize a word or phrase, or to indicate a reaction without saying anything. It is ironic that people will say, "She is beautiful," and while enunciating the word "beautiful," form an ugly frown.

Here is a game that is fun and that might help you remember not to frown when you are talking. Try saying the following sentence: "I don't have to frown." As you say the words, keep your face as frown-free as possible. See if you can do it! Try it several times, and soon you will become conscious of forehead wrinkling in yourself and in others. That will be the first big step in overcoming the grimace-frown habit, a habit that can be broken far more easily than you think.

The exercises in this book will help you break all of your skin-aging bad habits. When you learn to keep your forehead still and smooth, and when you combine that skill with face-building exercises, you will be able to stop further wrinkling and to make your present wrinkles disappear.

Nature is working for you; she is your friend and "on your side." Help her to help you. Only the very elderly, those who are extremely thin, or who have spent a lifetime in the sun and wind might have difficulty in erasing forehead lines. But most people will be amazed at the marked improvement in as little as two or three weeks. One of my pupils succeeded in smoothing her forehead completely in only two weeks. She explained, "Do you know I haven't frowned even once since you told me I didn't have to."

Now I'm telling you, all the readers of this book: "You don't have to!"

Stopping and Reversing the Aging of the Skin Through Facial Exercise

The skin is composed of many layers of cells, including fat cells that form a soft cushion and make the skin smooth and glowing. This skin is attached to the muscles by delicate connective tissue. In the young skin the connective tissue is strong and makes a secure bond between the muscles and skin surface.

When you drag or stretch your skin, if you habitually pull and toy with it, you weaken the connective tissue and stretch the skin. Harsh or forceful pressure on the skin, as well as stretching, can damage the delicate, fat globule-like cells and harm the texture of the face.

"But I never 'hurt' my skin!" you might protest. Don't you? Improper or rough washing and drying can be brutal treatment for facial skin.

Exercising the face is quite different from rubbing or moving the skin. When you exercise your face, you will be moving the skin and muscles in *unison*. They will be working together as one unit. This is a way of strengthening the tie between them, and of keeping the skin and muscles united as in youth.

So, do not be afraid of stretching the skin *and* muscles together. All the exercises in this book are designed to stretch the skin *with* the underlying muscles. The detailed directions will help you exercise the firm-toning way. Follow the directions carefully.

Here is an added plus: exercising muscles and skin will bring a vigorous blood supply to the surface of the skin, and you will enjoy a healthier, more vibrant complexion as well as toning and firming the facial contours.

The best way to restore skin and re-form facial contour, once the face has begun to sag, is through exercise. And, it is the only *natural* way. The life-giving blood—carrying vital oxygen and nutrients for the growing muscle tissue, and also carrying away wasted, used, old, or damaged cells, or impurities—is encouraged by exercise. The better the blood supply, the stronger the walls of the veins and capillaries, and the faster and more easily the muscles can be firmed and amplified. All the facial tissues benefit: skin, gums, muscles, veins, and, yes—even the rest of the body.

The Muscles of the Face

The picture shows the muscles of your face. These elastic tissues are beneath your skin.

Examine your face carefully. Are there any places where the muscles seem less vibrant and elastic? Are there parts of the cheeks that seem shrunken with hollows, shadows, and little pouches? Are these pouches beginning to form at either side of the chin, or at the corners of the mouth?

To restore firm facial contours and the healthy vigorous look of youth often takes several months of faithful practice. In those days and weeks of massage and exercise, you are reversing years of damaging forces. Do not expect immediate results in one or two days, but be confident that you can achieve visible, long-lasting results. You can improve not only the look, touch, color, texture, and vitality of your face and skin, but also your general health through the increased blood circulation and enhanced feeling of well-being that come from a carefully planned program of exercise.

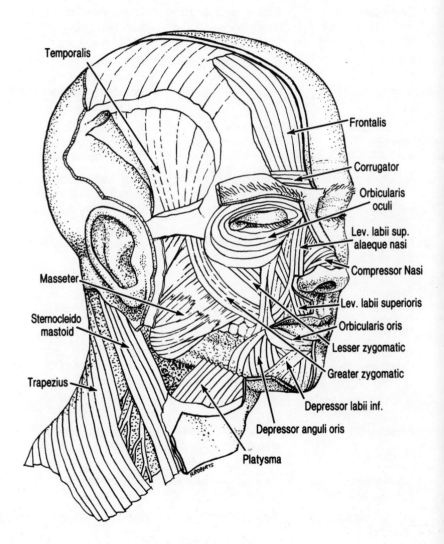

Temporalis

Frontalis

Corrugator

Orbicularis oculi

Lev. labii sup. alaeque nasi

Compressor Nasi

Masseter

Lev. labii superioris

Sternocleido mastoid

Orbicularis oris

Lesser zygomatic

Greater zygomatic

Trapezius

Depressor labii inf.

Depressor anguli oris

Platysma

7

Muscles of the Face

MUSCLE	Position	Function
Trapezius	Back of neck and shoulders	Draws shoulders together, pulls head back
Platysma	Main muscle from chin to chest	Pulls down corners of mouth; maintains contour of the neck
Sternocleido Mastoid	Runs obliquely along side of neck	Flexes head sideways, each side turning face to opposite side
Lesser Zygomatic	From molar bone to upper lip	Draws up side of mouth and upper lip; a laughing muscle
Greater Zygomatic	From cheekbone diagonally to angle of mouth	A laughing muscle
Temporalis	From temporal bone to inner side of jaws	One of the chewing muscles
Frontalis	Across the brow	Raises brow and wrinkles forehead
Orbicularis Oris	Circular muscle of the mouth	Main muscle of the mouth. Controls the upper and lower lips
Masseter	From cheekbone to outer side of lower jaw	Chewing muscle
Levator Labii Superioris	Runs across the cheek to the upper lip	Elevates upper lip
Depressor Labii Inferioris	Side of lower jaw	Elevates chin
Compressor Nasi	Outer lower border of bridge of nose	Compresses nostrils
Corrugator	A small muscle between the eyebrows	Controls the movement of the eyebrows

When you massage and exercise your face and neck, you will be moving the muscles, relaxing the muscles, tightening the muscles, flexing the muscles, and making the muscles grow strong, firm, and elastic. The massage and exercise will encourage a vibrant and youthful skin. They will retard and erase the effects of the years, the weather, gravity, your own bad habits, and even the sun.

If you examine the illustration, you'll see that muscles weave over the bones of your face and form a support for your jaw and other movable bones, for joints, and for the important sensory organs that are located on your face. The exercises in this book do not always follow the exact pattern of the facial muscles. They cannot, because the muscles weave in and out, over and under each other; they cross and recross with the thin anchors—the tendons—closing the net.

The massages and exercises presented here stretch and relax the arteries, veins, lymphatic system, and nerves as well as the muscles. The growth of strong, resilient, elastic muscles and glowing soft skin depends on the total development of the entire face. Massage and exercise work on everything, together.

When Should You Exercise?

Face-firming exercises can be done any time—morning, afternoon, or evening. It is best to exercise when you are least fatigued. Also it is good to rest after exercising. Many people find that the late afternoon is convenient: they are not too tired then, but still are ready for a very short (15- to 20-minute) nap after exercising. Then they arise completely refreshed, smooth, and ready for the evening's activities.

For some people exercising before retiring is a form of relaxation ritual that they enjoy. Then, off to bed to let the blood circulate and the sensory nerves in the face relax and grow strong while the soothing, peaceful sleep distributes youth-giving nutrients to the developing muscles.

You should never exercise when your face is tired; if your muscles feel rubbery, or quivery, stop immediately.

Magic Mineral Water Spray

You can make a magic fountain of youth that you can use in your own home or carry with you. The fountain of youth is simply a mineral water spray!

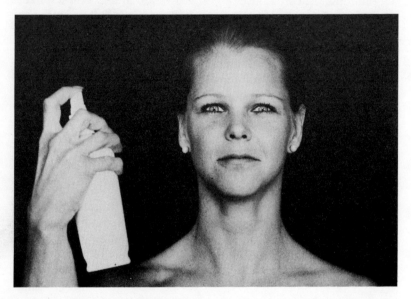

Here is how to make it:

1. Sterilize glass spray bottle by boiling it in water for about ten minutes. It is very important that the bottle be of glass rather than metal or any other material.
2. Mix a pint of mineral water (Mountain Valley*) with 1 teaspoon of apple cider vinegar.
3. Fill your spray bottle with the mixture and seal securely.

After spraying, *do not* dry your face. Apply your favorite moisturizer to the mist-wet face, and over that apply a protein cream, listed in the back of the book. Spray at least three times a day. You can carry the bottle with you and spray morning, afternoon, evening, on top of your makeup if you wish.

*I have used Mountain Valley Water for years and I feel it is the best for skin care. It comes from a spring deep beneath a huge marble bed.

Creaming Your Face

Most of the exercises require that your face be covered with a lavish coat of cream.

The cream around the mouth should be applied outward from the middle of the lip toward the ear. The cream under the eyes should be spread inward, from the lower outer eye toward the nose.

When you cream around the eyes, stop just short of the lashes, with slightly less cream on the upper eyelid than on the lower lid. Be sure the cream extends well past the eye area toward the temple. Cream carefully; the oil in the cream may make the eyes sting.

Don't forget the neck. When applying the cream to your neck, tip your head upward, tensing the neck muscles. Start the cream at the edge of the collarbone, then the cream should be moved upward and outward. Bring the cream over your entire cheek up to the ear. Cover the earlobe and under the lobe as well. The back of the neck should be creamed also.

The cream should be heavy enough to lubricate the skin thoroughly, and the skin might feel very slick to the touch. If you find it necessary, you can wear clean white cotton gloves on your hands when massaging your face. This will facilitate the firm hold on the muscle tissue and avoid slip-and-drag which could stretch the skin. When the exercise *requires* a lavish coat of cream, it is very important that you cream.

Taping the Forehead
(Your Forehead Head-Band)

There will be times when tape is applied before exercising. Before applying the tape, be sure that your face is carefully sprayed with mineral water to be moistened and covered with a protein-rich cream. Remember that a mineral water spray always goes first.

There will be several exercises to help you develop your frontalis muscle and smooth away the lines between your eyes and across your forehead. After completing your forehead exercises, you should tape your forehead. I call this method my "Forehead

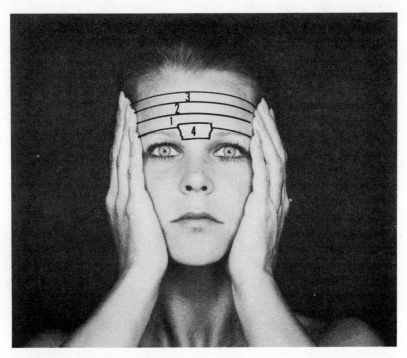

Head-Band." The taping acts as a wonderful reminder not to gesture or scowl with your forehead and also prevents additional lines from forming above your eyebrows.

You will need a roll of ¾″ surgical tape, called micropore surgical tape. This tape can be found in most pharmacies, but if you cannot get it, use "Band-Aid Clear Tape" made by Johnson & Johnson. Each person should find the tape that is most compatible with his or her skin. If you prefer not to use tape, you can make the head-band using moleskin wrap. Moleskin can be found in most drugstores, usually in the area that displays foot-care products. The head-band should be about 2 inches wide and securely anchored with an elastic bridge at the back. The band must fit snugly when placed above the brows.

Apply one layer of the tape directly over the eyebrows from one temple to the other. The second layer of tape should overlap the first by about ¼ inch, and the third layer about ¼ inch over the second. The fourth layer, between eyebrows, is about half the length of the first. As you become familiar with the tape process, you'll be able to measure the right amount of tape and apply it smoothly. It is important that the tape be firm and smooth and that it cover the wrinkled section of the forehead, but it should not extend to the hairline or pull or damage the hair in any way.

In addition to being applied directly after exercising the forehead, the Forehead Head-Band of tape can also be used after general facial exercises, or when you are relaxing at home, in private, at any time. It is an excellent reminder: no scowls or grimaces. If possible, leave the tape in place for approximately an hour after each application.

Removing the tape carefully is just as important as applying it correctly. Lift the tape from the edges at the temples. As you pull the tape off with one hand, keep the fingers on the other hand at the very edge of the still-sticking tape nearest the fingers. This will avoid any unnecessary pulling of the skin, and also reduce discomfort in removing the tape.

Moleskin may also be used in other areas of the face — between the eyes to avoid lines, or at the corners of the mouth.

General Suggestions for Exercises

The directions for each exercise must be exactly followed at every single practice. Success depends entirely on your doing the exercises correctly. An occasional error or lapse will not completely retard or reverse good results, but to skip any exercise in the program, or to practice incorrectly for several days, would mean a loss of nearly all the muscle control and smoothing gained.

The exercises should be done once or twice daily for at least three months for outstanding results. After these results are obtained, the muscles will be strong and elastic. Once the muscles are toned properly, the exercises can be omitted for a week or two at a time, every three or four months, with no harm. Or, a maintenance program of every other day can be sufficient to keep your face and neck at their firmest and smoothest.

If it is difficult for you to find a period of time long enough, you can, if you wish, divide the exercises into two or three short, 5-minute sessions. These mini-sessions can be at any time that is best for you.

Important:

1. Some lines and wrinkles may seem to be accentuated while you are doing the exercises. *A good cream covering before exercising will prevent any temporary lines from taking permanent hold.* Remember that this special program has been used by thousands and the exercises do not aggravate any skin problems.

2. Notice that many facial exercises also exercise the muscles of the neck and vice versa. This is an additional benefit. Another added benefit will be better posture and a more graceful carriage.

3. If on some days your face seems more lined or saggier than usual, it may mean that you have overstrained your facial muscles. This will not permanently harm them; a short rest will restore muscle tone. Skip your exercises for one day; if you look better the following day you can continue. If necessary, skip two or more days until your tired muscles recuperate.

4. Mother Nature works slowly — but surely. My experience with thousands of students helps me to estimate the exact time needed for any "lift" or any specific results. Exercising as a preventive measure need be done only occasionally; erasing deep lines requires a longer time.

As you look through this book, you'll notice that each exercise focuses on only one or two facial problems. In studying your own face in the mirror, you may find a concentration of problems — wrinkling and sagging of the skin, for example. I've tried to deal with one problem at a time; happily, solving that problem often brings a bonus of smoother skin in other facial areas.

Fifteen minutes is all you need — one quarter of an hour — about the same time it takes to put on your makeup. Naturally, in the beginning only one or two exercises will consume the allotted time. But gradually, as you memorize each movement, you'll find the complete basic program can be accomplished in less time than you thought possible! And then you are ready for the "special exercises." You can select only the exercises that will solve your special facial flaws, or you can go through all of the exercises for total facial firmness.

The old adage "practice makes perfect" is certainly true of exercise. The first few times you attempt a new exercise you may doubt whether you are doing it correctly or you may be concerned that it takes you a long time. Do you remember learning to drive a car? The actions that seem so automatic now were all somewhat awkward and time-consuming then. Facial exercise may be the same way: suddenly, and quite soon, you'll be smoothly and quickly completing the entire program in only 15 minutes a day.

Do not expect to master the complete program in one day, or even one week; but in less time than you might think, changes will appear! Each exercise includes an explanation of *how* and *why*. Logic will tell you there are no miracles, but your mirror will defy logic in a short period of time, if you follow these basic rules:

1. Exercise at least once a day. Twice a day is better.
2. Always use a mineral water spray before applying your pre-exercise lubricating cream.
3. Always apply a good lubricating cream before exercising. (Where indicated.) The cream should carefully and thickly cover the delicate eye area, but it need not cover the lids so heavily that it gets into your eyes. The cream should be left on the face during the entire 15 or more minutes of exercise. If you use more than the allocated time, let the cream remain on your face during those additional minutes.
4. Be sure that your face is absolutely clean before you start exercising. Use the cleansing cream, soap and water, or any combination of cleansers that works well for you. After the cleansing, spray with mineral water, and then apply a moisturizer to your still damp face. Then, over the moisturizer, a heavier cream. Apply the cream smoothly so that the entire face and neck area is covered. A thick coating of cream will keep your face well lubricated; if it is carefully washed away, it will not clog your pores.
5. Always use a mirror — at least until you have memorized each movement and are confident you are doing it correctly.
6. Breathe naturally in all exercises, unless the directions say otherwise.
7. After each exercise is completed, relax your face completely. Be sure the "worked" muscles are completely at rest.
8. Concentrate on the section of your face that is being exercised. Your mind as well as your muscles is needed. Clear your thoughts while exercising and you'll be delighted at how emotionally relaxed as well as physically toned you will be.
9. Slow and careful movements are best. *Faster* results can be seen from *slower* exercise movements. The same principles apply to facial exercises as to muscular exercises in other parts of your

body. Concentrating with your total attention on every action will make for faster results than hurriedly done or careless activity, even if it is repeated often. "Slow and steady *firms the face*."

10. During the first week or two of the program do not exercise too vigorously. The muscles and skin build slowly; as in other types of exercise, your goal is to build and strengthen, not damage any tissue.

11. You will find that it is helpful to read the directions for each exercise as you practice. You should also scrutinize the position of your hands and your features in a mirror as you follow each direction. You will probably find it necessary to read the directions for several weeks until they are memorized. Even after you are familiar with every movement, it is a good idea to recheck your hand and face-muscle positions from time to time.

12. Some exercises require a resistance or counterforce. This should be strong, firm, and slow, as indicated in the directions. Think of your facial muscles as elastic ribbons; pull them gradually without jerking or tearing.

PART TWO

The Basic Program

The following twelve simple facial exercises comprise the *Basic Program*, a program that has been carefully designed so that you can enjoy the fastest and most dramatic firming of your skin and facial muscles.

By faithfully exercising, you will not only change the contours of your face but keep the muscles, tissues, and skin soft, pliable, and resilient. How much improvement will the exercises bring? That obviously varies; no two people are the same, and the response of their skins to any program cannot be accurately predicted. But you can expect dramatic results — very soon. Some exercises, if done correctly, can bring results in a week. This is true mostly in the forehead area; the crow's feet — the small "smile lines" that spread from the outer corners of your eyes over your cheeks — also respond quickly. The muscles of the cheek are more difficult to affect.

It is perfectly normal for the muscles on one side of your face to be stronger than those on the other side; it is similar to right- and left-handedness — the stronger muscles work more easily and so respond to exercise and massage more quickly. But keep working at the weaker muscles. They, too, will respond and become firm and strong.

Go through the entire program for 15 minutes each day. Or, mix and match, working double time on the areas, wrinkles, or sags that are your own personal targets or goals. Consistency, carefully following the directions, and creaming — or not creaming as indicated — are most important.

And now for your 15-minute-a-day lift — up, up, and away!

15-Minute-A-Day Program

Exercise	Time
Developing the Frontalis Muscle (smoothing the forehead)	2 min.
Developing the Corrugator Muscle (smoothing the front)	1 min.
Developing the Temporalis Muscle (smoothing the temples)	2 min.
Rounding Out Hollow Cheeks	1 min.
Firming and Preventing Flabby Eyelids	1 min.
Strengthening and Smoothing the Muscles of the Eyelids	1 min.
Erasing Lines at the Corners of the Eyes and Under the Eyes	1 min.
Lifting and Toning All the Muscles around the Eyes	1 min.
Shaping the Lips	1 min.
Erasing Lines at the Sides of the Mouth; Raising Drooping Corners of the Mouth	1 min.
Removing a Double Chin	2 min.
Tightening a Double Chin	1 min.

If you want to do the following three exercises without creaming your face, do these exercises first. *These no-cream exercises are the only exception to the creaming rule.* But even with these exercises, be sure you use cream around your eyes. After completing these, apply cream over the rest of your face and neck and proceed with the other exercises.

Developing the Frontalis Muscle and Smoothing the Forehead

(No cream needed—2 minutes)

To smooth out the lines across your forehead you will have to develop the frontalis muscle. To do this you will massage the muscle using the balls of both hands. The balls are the fleshy pads between the thumb and wrist.

There are three variations to this exercise. Some people prefer one and some another. They all smooth those eyebrow wrinkles and frown lines, so use the one that suits you best!

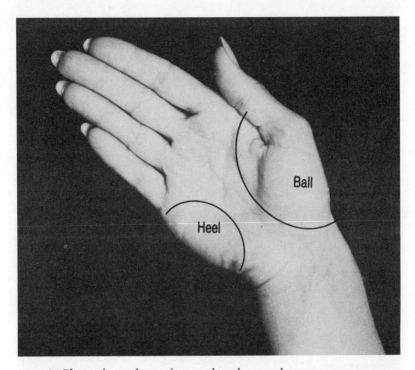

Ball

Heel

1. Place the palms of your hands together so you see your thumbs. Put the "praying hands" firmly against the middle of your forehead directly above your nose. Massage the muscle at the center of your forehead by slightly raising and lowering one hand, then the other.

As one hand goes up, pull the other down. The hands should now move only a little. Massage firmly, but not too vigorously. Do not let your hands slip over the skin; the idea is to move the muscle under the skin while stretching the skin as little as possible.

Move the rubbing palms with balls resting first to one side of the forehead — over the eyebrow, then the temple — then across to the other side. Massage continuously. Work hand back over forehead three times. Each pass over the entire forehead should take no more than a minute or two. Repeat the exercise two or three times, each side of the forehead.

Use this exercise several times a day for several weeks. You will notice an improvement in a few weeks — then adjust the number of times a day you exercise for maintenance.

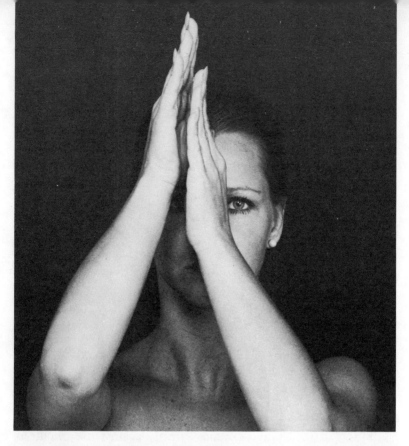

2. Place one hand, on each side of the forehead, ball section down, in the center of your forehead. The side of the hand, just below the thumb, should be held firmly against the forehead. Hold the skin tightly.

With the other hand, massage the section of the muscle on that side of the face. If you hold the skin firmly with the right hand, use the ball of the left for the massage. Work in a circular motion: up, around, back, and up again. Do not let the skin slip; hold firmly with the hand that is not massaging. Work from the center toward the temple. Reverse hands, so that the opposite hand holds and the other massages. Massage each side — center to temple, over the end of the eyebrow — two or three times.

3. In this variation the entire lower part of the palm of one hand will hold the skin of the forehead while the other hand does the massaging, using a circular motion away from the face, toward the hair. Press the palm firmly to the side of the head and don't allow the skin to slip. Hold the skin and muscles firmly as you work. Always massage or exercise from the center of the face toward the side. Massage both sides of the face.

Note: You can use your fingertips to do the massaging in variations 1, 2, and 3. If you do, be careful to apply the same firm, even pressure with all your fingers.

Developing the Corrugator Muscle and Smoothing a Frown
(No cream needed—1 minute)

This exercise will strengthen the little muscle between the eyebrows. The exercising of this muscle can smooth an angry frown. The muscle, called the "corrugator," has small but long thin fibers that cross the eyebrows and extend as far as the temples. When this muscle weakens, it can produce small lines near the temples and crow's-feet at the outer corners of the eyes.

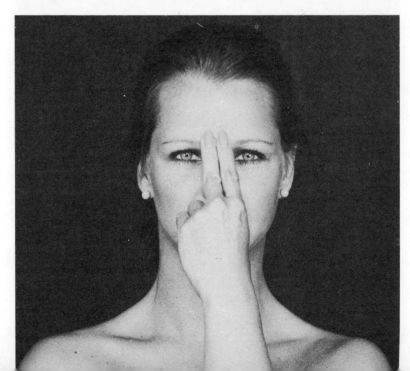

To erase the vertical lines that show on either side of the inner brows, above the nose — the corrugations — place the tips of the second and third fingers on the corrugation lines. Using both hands, you can exercise both sides of the face at the same time.

Press the tips of the fingers firmly against the skin. You will be able to feel the hard bone beneath the skin and thin layer of muscle. Holding firmly, massage up and down for a few moments, perhaps one-half of a minute. Then, horizontally massage, back and forth toward the temples. Then, work diagonally from upper temple, moving in the direction of the earlobe, or jaw. Massage in every direction for a moment or two. Then, back and forth once again, but move your finger in every direction, like the spokes of a wheel.

Finally, press the two fingers of each hand, once more, against the corrugator muscle, directly over the frown lines, and massage firmly, working the muscle in a circular motion, around and around.

Note: This exercise can be done with the tip of only one finger, but take care to hold the skin firmly, and do not dig your nails into the sensitive skin between the brows.

Developing the Temporalis Muscle and Smoothing the Temples
(No cream needed—2 minutes)

The most important exercise for the 15-minute face lift is the exercise that will develop the temporal muscle. This important muscle, located on the upper part of each side of your face, at the temples, is the master muscle in holding the side of your face smoothly and firmly.

In the young these temporal muscles are strong. The little muscle fibers pull back and up and keep the other facial muscles in place. Gravity, age, stretching, lack of the right kind of exercise, all of these factors work against this important facial anchor. And as one grows older, the temporal muscle (like other muscles) loses its elasticity and the entire face sags; the skin seems to droop and the marks of age are apparent. It is essential to keep this muscle vibrant and strong. The following group of exercises and variations can redevelop a weakened muscle and keep a firm muscle in good condition.

If you would like to see how the exercises for this muscle can rejuvenate your entire face, just place the heels of your hands on either side of your face at the outside of your cheekbone. Pull gently up and backward toward your temples. This is the action of a firm, strong temporal muscle: notice the "life" your entire face enjoys.

A moment's thought: the temporal muscle is the most important muscle for fast face-building, but it is also one of the most difficult to control. The temporal muscle *can* be mastered if you will be persistent in your efforts, and keep at it. Think of the muscle as a fanlike shape, between the eye and the upper edge of your ear. Strengthen the fan, and firm your entire face.

1. This is the basic exercise. It can be done with either the fingertips or the flat lower palm of each hand. If you use your fingertips, hold the four tips firmly together to form a pad. You will be working with both hands and firming both temporal muscles at the same time. Place the fingers or the flat of the hand firmly on the temple on each side of your face. The pressure should be directly over the fan-shaped muscle.

Place your teeth together in a firm bite and flex your jaw and temporal muscles so that they are hard. Without letting your hand slip, force your temporal muscles to move in a circular motion. Exercise the muscles by moving them upward, backward, downward, and around and forward toward the middle of the face, then around again, making a full circle. Make three full rotations of the muscle without allowing the skin to slip. Be sure that the muscle beneath the skin is benefiting from the exercise. Repeat the exercise three times a day for several weeks.

Note: The number of rotations of the muscle may later be increased or decreased, according to the results of this basic program.

2. The temporal muscle can be developed still further using this variation. Place your fingertips lightly on the temporal muscle. Your fingers will be feeling the movement of the muscle, but will not be moving the muscle. Open your mouth very wide so that it forms a large letter "O." Work your jaws back and forth in a chewing motion, but only close your jaw about an inch. Your mouth should be open — partially, then widely — through this entire exercise. Open and partially shut your jaws ten to twenty times.

You should be able to feel the movement of your jaws through a flexing of your temporal muscle. Do you feel the movement of the muscle under your fingertips? You should!

3. The last variation of the temporal-firming exercise is the most difficult because it requires great concentration in the beginning. With this exercise you can learn to control and activate the two temporal muscles through mental control. You will be able to move these muscles up and back at *will*. And, as you move these muscles, they will become stronger and actually activate other muscles in the face. You will be "thinking" them in place.

Close your eyes and imagine that there is a pulling backward and upward of all the muscles and skin around your eyes, ears, and temples. Concentrate until you can actually feel the pulling of these temporal muscles. It might help to imagine that you can move your ears and flatten them back against your head. Practice this effort and hold the tensed muscles as long as possible.

Practice as often as possible, at spare moments, during the day and in the evening. You can do it anywhere, anytime. The control of the temporal is a physical process that comes from mental will and concentration. When you do master these important muscles, you will have accomplished a great deal, and you will be rewarded by facial tone and firm-textured skin that will roll back years.

These three exercises you have just learned — developing the frontalis muscle to keep your forehead smooth, developing the corrugator muscle to banish frowns and that ugly scowling look, and developing the temporal muscles to firm your entire face — are all basic to the 15-minute face lift. If you practice faithfully, in a short time you will be delighted with the results that will be reflected in your mirror. Gradually, as you become adept, the exercises can be done in a shorter period of time. Then you should add new routines to your daily exercise program.

Note: These next exercises can be done only when your face is creamed; review the directions for creaming your face.

Rounding Out Hollow Cheeks

(Cream needed—1 minute)

This exercise should be done as *slowly* as possible.

When the mouth is drawn to the right, the pull is on the left cheek muscle; the mouth drawn to the left pulls the right cheek. The jaw will move with the mouth. The teeth need not be clenched or even entirely shut.

Lightly close the lips.

Pucker and purse the lips.

Pull the pursed mouth as far as possible to the right.

Creating a suction in your mouth, pull the left cheek tightly over the molars and pull the flesh of the left cheek slowly over the teeth toward the right. (Remember to make each movement as firm and slow as possible.)

Relax the mouth. Now pucker and pull the mouth to the left using the same actions as you did on the right side.

Repeat, pulling the mouth to each side three times. (If you have very deep cheek hollows or a very thin face, repeat this exercise five or six times for each side.)

Note: Your face may not look exactly like the picture; every face and face shape is different. The picture is only a general guide, but by studying it, you can adjust your action.

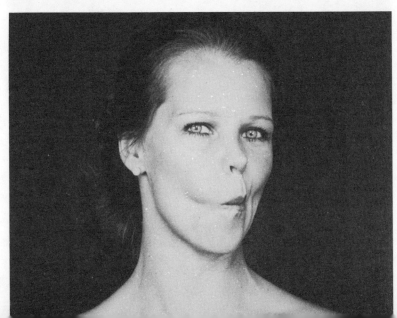

Firming and Preventing Flabby Eyelids
(Cream needed—1 minute)

Place four fingers of each hand over the eyelids.

Press the fingers firmly against the lower edge of the brow, just at the edge of the bone.

Attempt to close the eyelids, but resist the closing by raising the eyebrows sharply and strongly with each four fingers, as the eyes are being closed. In raising, draw the brows up firmly at the outer tips. This will exercise the muscle at the corner of each eye as well as exercising the eyelids.

Closing the eyelids against the pressure should be like a prolonged squint.

Close and resist to the count of six.

Relax. Allow hands to drop.

Repeat six times.

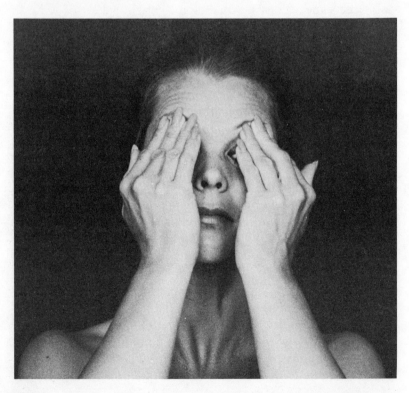

Strengthening and Smoothing the Muscles of the Eyelids
(Cream needed—1 minute)

Be sure the eyes, brows, and temples are thickly creamed. Place the first finger (index finger) of each hand on the outer corner of each eye. Place the second or middle finger under the eyebrow about an inch from the outer edge, over the highest point of the eyebrow arch.

Press firmly and hold as you draw the skin and the underlying muscle toward the temples. Move the flesh upward until the eyes seem to slant.

As you force the flesh upward, open and close the eyes six times. When you close your eyes, shut them tightly. You will feel the muscles pulling hard under your fingertips, but try not to allow the flesh to slip. The index finger will actually slip a tiny bit each time you close your eyes tightly, only because the lubricating cream will prevent a slip-free hold.

After six eye movements "open-shut," relax, rest, lowering your fingers. After you rest a moment or two, repeat the exercise, opening and shutting six times.

Repeat the exercise four times to make 24 winks of the eyes.

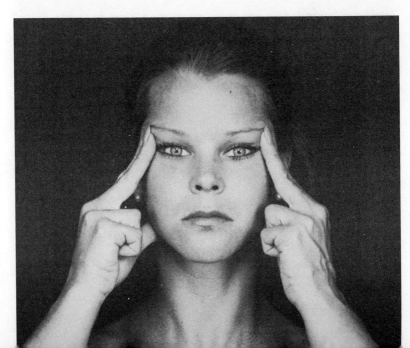

Erasing Lines at the Corners of the Eyes and Under the Eyes

(Cream needed—1 minute)

The muscles at the sides of the eyes are very close to the eyeball, so in doing this exercise place the fingers just at the outer edge of the eyes. Do not position the fingers over the lids or exert any pull on the eyelids; just the pressure of placing the finger on the delicate skin may draw it back a little (toward ears) as eyelids draw toward nose.

Place the index or middle finger or both fingers of each hand at the outer corner of the eye.

Try to gradually shut the eyelids tightly.

Resist the closing eyelid with firm but gentle pressure from the positioned finger. (In order to get a good pull on the muscle under the finger, you must shut the eyelids tightly, squinting.)

As the eyelids close and draw toward the nose, pull the fingers back slightly toward each ear. You will feel resistance of the pulling lid.

Hold for a count of five.

Relax, allow hands to drop.

Repeat squinting-pull six times.

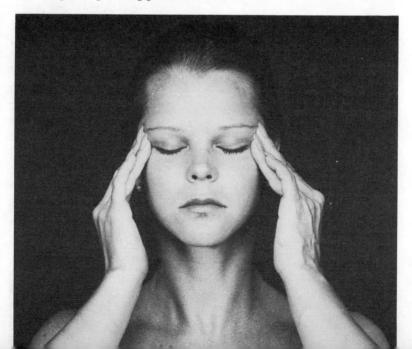

Lifting and Toning All the Muscles Around the Eyes

(Cream needed—1 minute)

Use both hands and be sure that the face and forehead are well covered with cream.

Place the fingers of each hand so the tips are lightly against the center of the forehead and parallel to the hairline and brows.

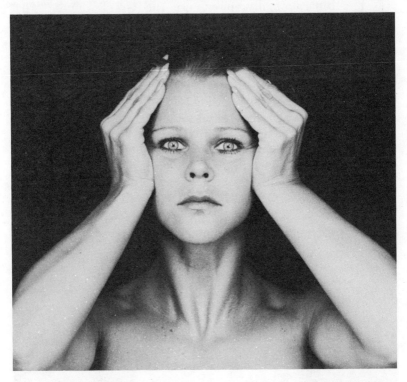

The balls of each hand should be below the eyes and just rest against the cheekbone on each side of the face.

Using a very soft and caressing motion, move the fingers outward and upward, while the balls of the hand press gently against the cheekbones and move the skin on the upper cheek.

The motion should be smooth, gentle, and lifting.

Repeat six times.

Shaping the Lips
(Cream needed—1 minute)

This is a three-part exercise that will plump and firm the lips and restore an even lip line. It also firms the muscle about the mouth and nose.

1. This part of the exercise is for flexibility of the lips and the muscles around the mouth and nose.

Breathing normally, pronounce the vowel sounds "Ah," "Oh," "Ee," and "Uh."

Repeat ten times.

2. This exercise will prevent small vertical lines from forming on the upper lip. It will also deepen and clarify the pretty indentation that runs between the nose and the upper lip, and improve the general shape of the lips.

Use an ample covering of cream on the upper lip.

Place the tip of the index finger in the cleft, or dent, at the center of the upper lip. The pad of the finger should be held securely just above the lip line.

Place the third finger (middle finger) of the same hand at the corner of one side of the mouth and the thumb at the other corner.

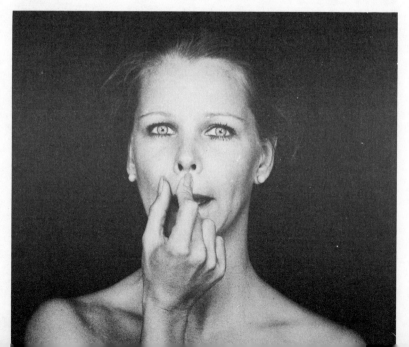

Draw the thumb and middle finger together, squeezing the flesh of the upper lip with a firm motion.

The thumb and middle finger should meet the index finger at the cleft of the upper lip. You may wish to hold your mouth open slightly so the bottom lip doesn't get pushed.

Repeat the action six times.

3. This exercise is for a lip that is already creased. Use an ample amount of cream on the upper lip and firm pressure when smoothing the wrinkles. Be careful not to stretch or pull the skin.

Note: Remember not to hold the mouth too tense. Relax, and try to keep the muscles on the upper lip soft and pliable.

Smile slightly so the upper lip is pulled against the upper teeth.

Repeat the exercise five times.

Erasing Lines at the Sides of the Mouth; Raising Drooping Corners of the Mouth
(Cream needed—1 minute)

For good results in this exercise, the jaws must be wide open when the lips are held over the teeth. The success of the action depends on the firming and stretching of the muscle around the mouth. This muscle must be flexed, firmed, and built to remove the drooping corners of the mouth or wrinkles around that area.

Open your mouth, keeping your lips as narrow as possible.

Pull your lips over the upper and lower teeth, but do not close your jaws. If you find it very difficult to hold your jaws open while forcing the lips over the teeth, it may be helpful to place your hand around your chin and hold your lower jaw down, while your lips are forced in. After you have practiced and your mouth and jaw muscles become stronger, you will be able to complete the motion without the aid of your hand.

Pull your lips together over the jaws and teeth so there is only enough opening to insert your little finger between your lips (your mouth should be positioned almost as if you were whistling). Or, it may be helpful to pretend that you are trying to whisper "Oh" with the front of your lips.

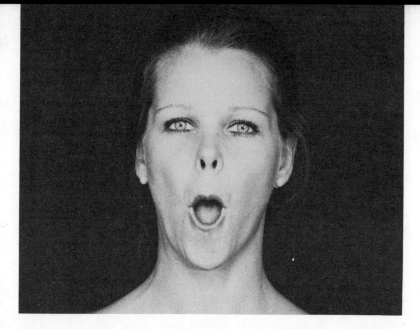

Take fifteen counts (mentally) while you are positioning your lips and pulling the lip muscles taut.

Hold lips in tight whistle position for five counts.

Repeat three times.

Removing a Double Chin

(Cream needed—2 minutes)

Cream your face and neck carefully before exercising.

Splash the face and neck with cold water for four or five minutes after these exercises.

This is a five-part exercise.

1. Bend the head backward until it rests on the middle back.

Contract the muscles in the front of your neck. Try to make them rigid and tense.

Close your teeth tightly. Clench your jaws until the cords of the neck stand out.

Open and close jaws five times.

2. With head still back, close jaws; keep teeth closed.

Raise your head to an upright position, while keeping your neck muscles tense.

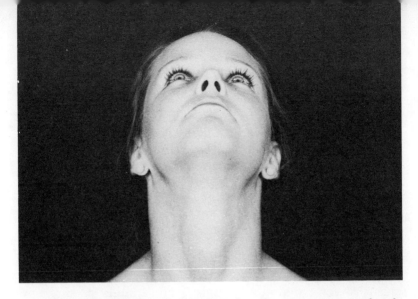

Push your head back, keeping chin down as you raise head.

3. Keep neck back, chin down.

Turn head to the left four times; then turn to the right four times.

Rest, relaxing neck muscles.

Repeat this exercise four times. In this way you will be turning the tensed neck muscles 16 times to the left and 16 times to the right.

4. Bend head backward, tense muscles.

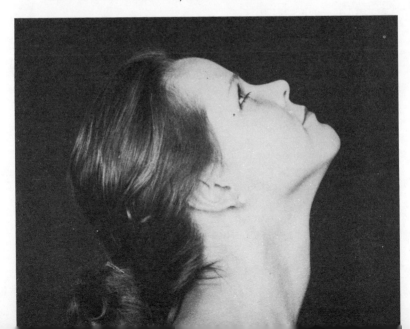

Pinch the tensed muscles of the double chin with the thumb and a doubled-over first finger.

Continue pinching until the fat is warm and the skin becomes red. (Pinch by holding the under-skin fat pad; do not pull the skin by pinching too much flesh at a time.)

5. Keeping your head back, bend the first finger until the first joint and second joint make right angles. You will be using the knuckle section for the next part of the exercise.

Following the line under the jaw, move the knuckles of the bent first finger from the center of the chin to the ear.

Do not pull or drag the skin; the effect should be a soothing massage.

Note: Keep the skin soft and pliable and well nourished with creams as you remove the fat pad. Careful stimulation and nourishment will prevent wrinkles as the double chin disappears.

Tightening a Double Chin

(Cream needed—1 minute)

Cream the neck carefully.

Place the fingertips of the right hand at the base of the neck, where the neck meets the shoulders, and directly under the chin.

Using a circular motion as shown in the illustration, move the hand to the right and upward until the fingers are under the right ear.

Bring the fingers down again in the same way to the base of the neck. Repeat five times.

Relax.

Using the same technique and circular motion, massage the left side of the neck from base to ear, and back.

Repeat five times.

Place the backs of the fingers, the knuckles, together under the chin.

Draw the knuckles soothingly up toward the ears. Stop under the earlobes.

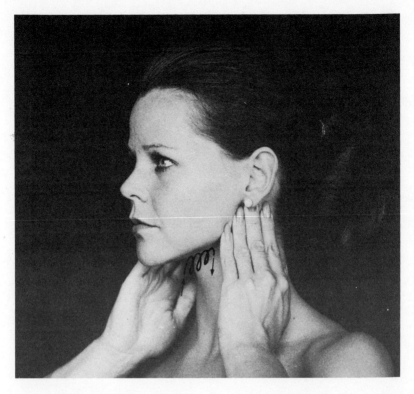

Repeat ten times.

After exercising, apply cold water to the neck, first in splashes and then with a soaked cloth held to the neck for about five minutes, to invigorate and stimulate the tissues.

The Basic Program is now yours: you can adapt it to your special needs or use it as a stay-firm preventive plan. Keep reviewing the exercises until you are comfortable with all of the movements. Check your finger positions in front of a mirror to be sure placement and motion will bring you the fastest results in the shortest time.

PART THREE

The Special Program

The next set of exercises is a supplement to the basic 15-minute face lift program. You can use any, or all, of these exercises in addition to the basic 15-minute program, or you can use only one of them for a beauty problem that is your own special target. These special exercises are aimed at specific flaws; if you use them in combination with the basic program, you will see fast and very dramatic results.

You can repeat these exercises once, twice, or many times each day; you can use any of them as a maintenance tool, exercising every other day or two or three times a week. Remember these are to be used *in addition* to the 15-minute basic program: they cannot be used *instead* of the basic program without vastly diminishing your total results.

You'll notice that these exercises do not include a specific time as did the exercises in the basic program. This is because you can use them as often as needed. But remember, the same rules for exercising and for creaming in Part Two are to be followed.

Erasing Lines on the Forehead
(No cream needed)

This exercise is intended both for horizontal lines from temple to temple and for vertical lines from brow to hairline. At first it will seem to encourage a vertical line between the brows, but the movement outward, toward the temples, will easily erase the first finger-induced creases.

When doing this exercise do not allow the fingers to slip, moving only the skin; the skin and undermuscle must be massaged with the same action.

Place the first three fingers of each hand together so the tips of each form a vertical pad. Place the tips in two rows at the center of the forehead.

The fingers of the right hand and left hand should be about ½-inch apart.

Press firmly; you can balance your fingertips by placing your thumbs gently against your hairline.

Move the fingers and the flesh beneath in the following way: right hand up, about ¼-inch; left hand down, about ¼-inch.

Reverse, pushing the left up and the right down and stretching and moving the skin and muscle on the forehead with fingers. The flesh will be pulled outward and diagonally.

Gradually move the right hand toward the right temple and the left hand toward the left temple, enlarging the space between the fingers.

Finish with an upward stroke toward the hairline.

Relax. Repeat this exercise a minimum of three times, always finishing with an upward stroke.

Note: This is not suggested if you have very long nails or the pads at the tips of your fingers allow your nails to touch the skin on your forehead.

Do not press on any tender spots on the outer edges of the forehead.

Smoothing Horizontal Lines Across the Forehead
(No cream needed)

Raise the eyebrows as high as possible, lifting the muscles of the forehead.

Holding the muscles in this position, place the right hand, palm down, firmly and flatly on the forehead. Secure the hold by pressing the flat palm of the hand against the forehead. Two hands may be used for extra grip. The hand or hands must be placed to cover the lower part of the forehead and both brows, as well as the center. The pulled muscles are now in a position to be exercised.

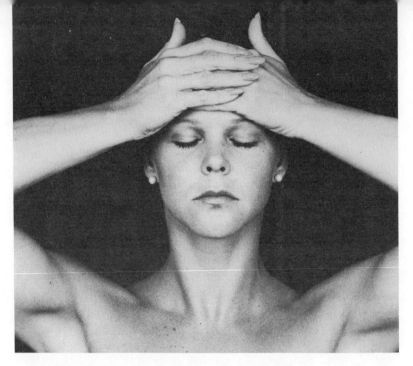

Close the eyes. Eyelids must be closed in order to exert the strongest downward muscle pull.

Concentrate on pulling downward with the forehead muscles. Draw these muscles down hard by pulling against the anchoring palms, which should resist this drawing and pulling down of the muscles.

Count to fifteen while pulling downward against the resistance.

Relax between repetitions, but you need not remove the hands.

Repeat six times for deep lines, three times for faint or slight lines.

Developing Tone and Firmness in Cheek Muscles and Cheeks

(Cream needed)

This is an excellent exercise for the entire face and a good general exercise.

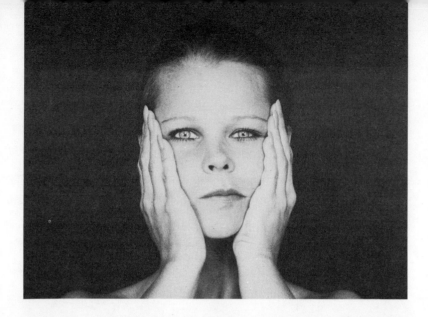

Place your hands on the sides of your face so that the outer edge of your hand, from your little finger to the bottom of the heel of your palm, is firmly against the skin of the outer portion of the face.

Holding the hands in this position, with your fingers pull the muscles under your eyes slightly upward, smoothing away any crow's-feet. With the heel of the hand pull outward and upward so that any flesh on the sides of the nose and any softness at the base of the nose are smoothed.

When the skin is held firmly and tightly, push the lips forward and slightly pucker them, as if you were about to say, "Oh!" When you hold your mouth in this way, the line from the nose to the mouth will be erased.

Hold the cheeks taut with the balls of the hands and slowly pull the "Oh"-shaped lips first to one side of the face, then the other. Pull the lips as far to the side as possible. You will feel a strong pull on your cheek muscles as you point your lips to the other side.

Alternating sides, bring the lips right, then left, then right again. Repeat the action five times on each side.

Relax. Lower your hands and allow the face to regain its natural position.

Repeat the entire exercise twice. This will total ten mouth movements in each direction.

Smoothing the Lines from the Nose to the Mouth; Firming Sunken Muscles at the Corners of the Nose

(Cream needed)

Use plenty of cream so that the fingers slip smoothly over the skin.

If any teeth are missing, they must be replaced before this exercise can be effective.

The lines from the corners of the mouth to the base of the nose are often the first to form. They have an aging effect on even a young face. The first movement of this two-part exercise should be light and soothing; the second should be firm and pressured.

Place the middle finger of each hand at the corner of the mouth.

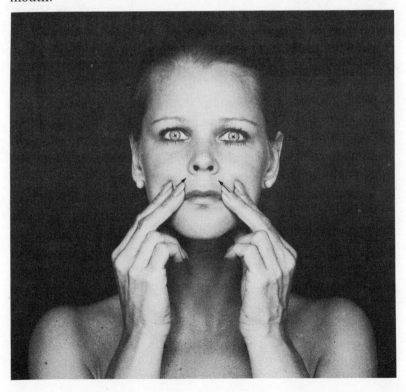

Very gently push and work the pads of the fingers upward to the base of the nose. Follow and press along the lines of the wrinkle which often forms between the nose and the corner of the mouth. Be sure that you are pressing the skin and the muscle together and you are not dragging the skin alone.

Then place all the fingers along the line. With a strong, heavy pressure pull all the fingers across the cheeks toward the top of the ears. Pull tautly. This stretches and works the muscle at the base of the nose.

Repeat both parts of this exercise six times.

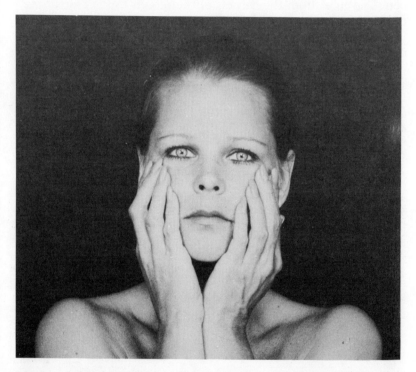

Note: If there are lines in the cheeks near the lips, use the same two-part approach: just a soothing motion upward and then a firm pressure on the cheeks moving toward the top of the ears.

Developing Muscles over the Bridge of the Nose; Strengthening the Muscles at the Inner Corners of the Eyes
(Cream needed)

Be sure that your face has been sprayed with mineral water and then thickly creamed, especially the eye area. You may want to use gloves for this exercise.

Place the middle finger of the left hand over the skin between the eyebrows. The fingertip should be pointing to the right.

Place middle finger of the right hand over the bridge of the nose next to the inner corner of the left eye. You can gently hook your finger around the bridge of your nose; if your nose has a high bridge it will be an excellent anchor.

Pull the skin and muscle under the left finger to the left. Pull the skin and muscle at the inner corner of the left eye up over the bridge of the nose toward the right.

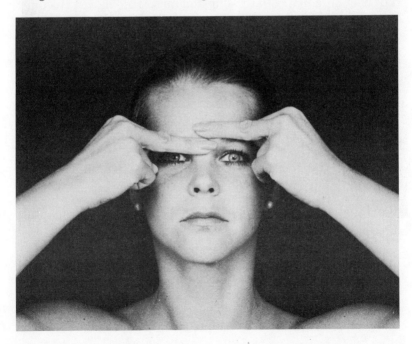

Relax and repeat this double motion five times.

Reverse the hand positions so that the middle finger of the right hand is between the eyebrows and pointing to the left, and the middle finger of the left hand is over the bridge of the nose and at the inner corner of the right eye. Repeat the motion five times.

Reapply cream if needed.

Using the middle fingers of both hands, smoothly press the wrinkles between the brows with a firm but gentle upward stroke.

In this second part of the exercise the lower finger (the ring finger) will move more than the upper finger (the index finger). The upper finger, placed directly over the lined area between the brows, should remain almost stationary. It must be held firmly and provide resistance for the pulling action of the lower finger.

Use a firm motion when the line between the brows is deep, a light surface movement for a faint line. The flesh — skin and muscle — should be twisted and stretched between the two firmly held fingers. Repeat this firm upward motion five times.

Note: Be sure that both the skin and muscle are moved as a unit; do not allow the holding finger between the brows to slip and drag only the skin.

It may seem that this exercise deepens the lines between the brows, but it actually develops the drawn-in underlying tissue and stimulates the muscles at the bridge of the nose.

Firming Sagging and Hollow Cheeks; Erasing Sagging from Nose to Mouth; Tightening Flabby Skin and Wrinkles in Front of Ears
(Cream needed)

Yawn, opening the mouth and jaws as wide as possible and forming the mouth into a long "O" shape. Then, open just a bit wider!

Slowly close the jaws, but as you do, try to resist the pulling muscles that close the mouth. Do not allow the molars at the back of the upper mouth to meet the molars of the lower jaw. Do this as slowly as possible. As you close your jaw you resist; close the mouth and jaw, fighting it.

When the teeth do finally meet, your muscles should be tense. Hold this tension a few seconds longer — count slowly to 25 in your mind; concentrate on keeping tension on the sides of the face. Relax the muscles very slowly and gradually.

Repeat three times. However, if your jaws or the muscles on the sides of your face ache, do not repeat. Try again tomorrow.

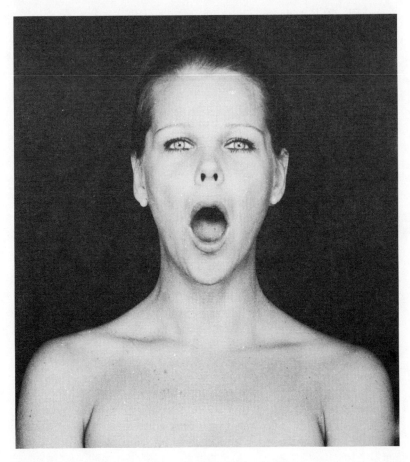

Note: This exercise cannot make your mouth wider, not even a trifle. The lips can be developed and filled out only through massage.

Strengthening the Muscles of the Eyes

(Cream needed)

This exercise strengthens the muscles and nerves of the eyes as well as the lids over and beneath the eyes. It also strengthens the muscles at the bridge of the nose. These have a tendency to draw in and make the nose look hawkish and the eyes too close together and deep-set.

This exercise is especially helpful in bringing the eyeball forward and retarding its tendency to sink back into the socket — one of the normal happenings in the aging process.

As you take a long deep breath through your nose, pull your upper lip down so that it covers the lower lip.

Hold the deep breath and open your eyes as wide as possible, focusing your sight intently on a spot or object in the far distance.

Concentrate on that object or spot until your facial muscles seem to enliven.

Your eyes will open even wider and your nostrils will automatically dilate. You will become aware of the stimulated muscles around your eyes.

Continue holding your breath; you will become very aware of stimulation around your eyes. Try to concentrate on the taut muscles in back of the eyes.

Do not turn your head, but moving only your eyeballs look to the right as far as possible, then to the left, then upward, then downward.

Roll your eyes around: far right, far left, up, and down.

Close your eyes tightly and exhale. Relax.

Repeat the exercise, reversing the direction of the eye — turning and rolling. Relax.

Repeat the exercise every day until you can roll your eyes, while holding your breath, five or six times with ease.

Note: Beware of doing this when you are over-tired. Your eye muscles may ache the first few times you exercise. This shows that the muscles are weak and need to be strengthened.

Variation: Inhale through your nose as you bring your upper lip down over your lower lip.

Holding your breath, open your eyes very wide and focus on a point directly in front of you.

Fix your gaze on this point for several seconds or until you become aware of a strong pulling sensation on the muscles of the back of the eyes.

Exhale and relax.

Repeat this exercise three times.

Note: Go through this exercise once the first day, twice the second, and so forth; increase to as many as five times a day, or as often as you are able to cream your face and exercise.

For a quick and easy eye-firming exercise that you can do any time and any place and without cream, simply open your eyes wide and look steadily at a fixed point. Repeat this easy-to-do exercise at least three times a day for fast results.

Erasing Crow's Feet; Smoothing Lines Beneath the Eyes
(Cream needed)

This is an excellent exercise for strengthening the muscles around the eyes, if they are beginning to lose tone. It is helpful for erasing wrinkles.

Check the position of the fingers and hands in your mirror before completing any of the exercise actions.

Be sure the sides of your face, especially the eyes, are well creamed. The mouth and cheeks must also be heavily lubricated.

Place the first finger, the index finger, of each hand on the large bone just in back of the ear.

The palm of each hand should firmly cradle the side of your face.

Position your little finger at the outer corner of each eye.

Push the flesh beneath the little finger upward and backward toward the hairline so that the muscles of the entire face are pulled upward and outward, toward the top of the ear and temple. Hold firmly.

Keeping the hands in this position, and the flesh taut, open your eyes very wide.

Push the lips forward in a slight pucker as though you were forming the "Oh" sound.

Keeping the lips in the circular shape, pull the mouth as far to the right as possible. Try to point the mouth toward the right earlobe.

Open your mouth and inhale.

Force the inhaled air to the right side of your cheek. (It will bulge the cheek slightly.)

Close your mouth for a moment, capturing the inhaled air in your right cheek.

Concentrate to be sure that your eyes are held wide open and your mouth is tightly closed when you force air into your cheeks. There should be a strong pull on the muscles at the outer corners of the eyes, as well as on the muscles on the upper cheeks.

Exhale, releasing the air, but keeping your hands in opposition, and the mouth to the right.

Repeat the inhalation two more times.

Return your mouth to the natural position. Lower your hands. Relax and rest to the slow count of five.

Repeat the complete exercise, drawing the mouth to the left, inhaling and opening and closing three times.

Relax and rest to the count of five.

Repeat the entire exercise three times, until you have opened the mouth, captured air, and closed your mouth for nine times on each side.

Smoothing Lines and Puffs under Eyes; Firming Bags and Sagging of Under-Lids
(Cream needed)

If this exercise is done correctly, many small wrinkles will form under the eyes, at the sides of the eyes, and at the sides of the eyelids. This wrinkling is only temporary. It cannot take permanent effect if you use plenty of cream around the eyes.

When creaming the eyes, do not apply the cream so close to the edge of the lid that the cream, liquifying on your skin, allows oil to get into your eye. The oil in any cream will be irritating to your eye.

Shut your eyes tightly. Contract your lids as much as possible.

Draw the muscles of the lid close together until they are tense.

Open the eyelids slowly and only the least little bit.

Keep the squinted position and the tension on your eyelids. Do not relax the muscles of the lids.

Open the eyelids as gradually and slowly as possible.

Count to fifteen as you slowly open your lids and tense the muscles with a pulling draw.

Relax the eyelids; open them widely, all the way.

Close the lids and repeat the exercise three times.

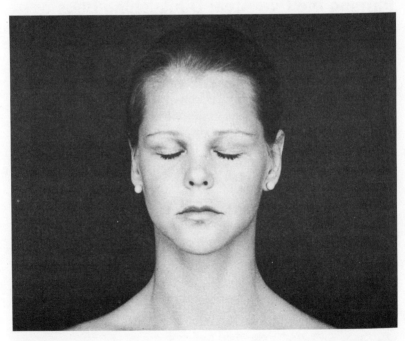

Note: As an extra precaution, press the area where wrinkles were formed by the exercise — the skin just under the eyes and at the sides of the eyes — gently with the tips of your fingers, three or four times, smoothing the skin in this area. The temporary wrinkles will vanish.

Erasing Curved Lines over Eyebrows
(No cream needed)

This exercise will not entirely erase vertical lines on your forehead; it is for curved lines.

Place the heel of your hand or hands firmly over the uncreamed lines.

Draw down on the muscles of the lined area of the forehead. Try to separate the forehead from the hairline. Pull down as hard as possible.

Hold for six counts; repeat six to ten times.

Firming the Eye Area; Diminishing Bags or Puffiness around Eyes
(Cream needed in eye area only)

Five exercises are given below; select all or any of the exercises that you wish. They all are effective in firming the eye area. Exercising the eyes also strengthens all the facial muscles.

Any sudden movement of the eyes or head can cause a feeling of dizziness. Omit these exercises if you are feeling any discomfort. Check with your doctor if you have any questions or concerns about your reaction to these exercises.

1. Close your eyes.

Roll eyeballs in a complete circle clockwise.

Repeat six times.

With eyes still closed, roll eyeballs in a complete circle counterclockwise.

Repeat six times.

Note: This eye-rolling exercise can be done most easily with the lids closed. However, if you prefer, you can do this, and other exercises, with your eyes open.

2. Close eyelids.

Raise eyebrows as high as possible, resisting with the eyes and lids.

Strain and hold for five counts. Relax.

Repeat three to six times.

3. Hold face forward without tilting throughout this exercise.

Move eyes slowly first to the right.

Hold for the count of six.

Move eyes back to forward position, then to the left. Hold for the count of six. Back to forward position.

Repeat three times to each side.

4. Hold face in forward natural position.

Look upward as far as possible without moving head.

Move eyes to the right, forward position, and then to the left. Hold for the count of six in each direction.

Repeat: up, right, left, forward position three times each.

Repeat same exercise for count of three with eyes moving down not up, then right, left, etc.

5. Open eyes wide.

Focus on a distant object.

Hold for count of five.

Repeat three or four times a day.

Any of the preceding five eyes exercises will be sufficient for daily exercising, but for interest you might want to alternate the exercises.

You may skip one day each week to rest eye muscles.

Erasing Crow's-Feet; Firming Dips and Sags at the Side of the Chin; Making Firm and Expressive Lips

(Cream needed)

The higher you can keep your eyebrows while doing these exercises, the better the results.

Hold the teeth firmly together while you are working on the lower part of the face.

Forming a tense smile, harden the muscles at the sides of your chin and under your chin. You should be able to feel the muscle tensed with your hand.

Stretch and broaden your lower lip; make the mouth as wide as possible. The lips may be slightly parted if that seems helpful.

Tense and stretch the muscles on the inside of the mouth and cheeks.

Elevate your eyebrows, pulling them up toward the hairline as far as possible.

Your entire face should be tense and stretched.

Hold for at least the count of 15, eventually working up to 25 seconds.

Relax your face.

Repeat three times.

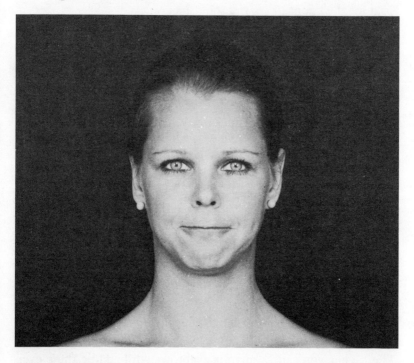

Note: Tensing the muscles on the sides of the chin before raising the eyebrows is easier than tensing all muscles at the same time.

Tightening the Sag from the Nose to the Mouth; Erasing the Lines at the Sides of the Mouth and on the Upper Lip

(Cream needed)

Open mouth to a vertical "O" position.

Close eyes.

Raise eyebrows as high as possible. If necessary, use your hands to hold the eyebrows in an elevated position.

Holding this position, attempt to close lips over the teeth of the open jaws. While holding the eyebrows up, close the lips, pulling them together over the teeth.

A pull should be felt in the middle of the face over the upper lip and middle section of the lower lip. The eyebrows must be kept elevated to create a pull-counterpull on the muscles.

Count to fifteen while closing the lips.

When lips are closed as much as the pull will allow without closing jaws, hold lips in steady position for five more counts.

Relax.

Repeat one to three times.

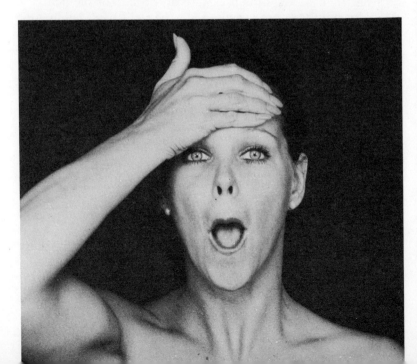

Firming Sagging Cheeks; Tightening and Smoothing Neck Muscles

(Cream needed)

It is important to have a strong pull on muscles of the neck to make this exercise most effective.

Place the fingers of the left hand across the left side of the face. The first finger should be on the large bone just behind the ear; the second, or middle, finger in the slight depression just in front of the ear. The third and fourth fingers, with the heel of the hand, on the side of the cheek.

Bend your head to the right. Do not change the position of the hand against the flesh of the cheek.

Firmly, push the entire hand upward. The flesh under the firmly held fingers will move upward against the bones of the face.

Drop the head slowly toward the chest.

Keep your hand firmly on the outer cheek with the flesh pushed upward.

Raise the head, flesh still held firmly and tightly upward.

Slowly bend the head backward over the right shoulder.

Now do the entire exercise with the right hand holding the right cheek, and the head bending to the left, repeating seven times.

Firming the Muscles of the Chin

(Cream needed)

This exercise will loosen the muscles around the lower jaw. It encourages good circulation in the skin through an increased blood supply.

Be sure you have an ample covering of cream so your fingers will move easily on the skin.

Place the middle finger of the right hand on the chin, just below the outer corner of the left side of the mouth.

Make circular motions across to the middle of the chin, as shown in the illustration, pushing the flesh firmly.

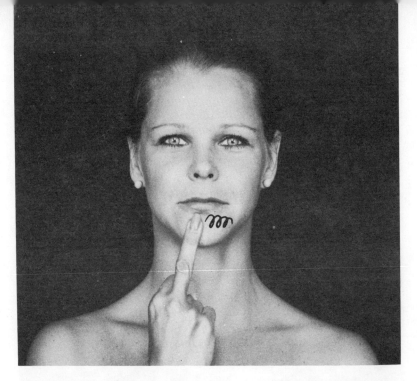

Without lifting the finger from the skin, dip the middle finger down, passing it under the chin.

In one firm sweep from under the chin, bring the massaging finger back to the middle of the chin.

Repeat ten times.

Reverse the motion, using the middle finger of the left hand to massage the right side of the chin.

Repeat ten times.

Erasing Lines under the Point of the Chin
(Cream needed)

For most people the exercises for the neck and chin just mentioned will remove lines. However, this additional exercise can be used by those who prefer it.

Cream the neck and face carefully.

Thrust the point of your chin out as far as possible.

Hold this position and pull your lower lip up as high and

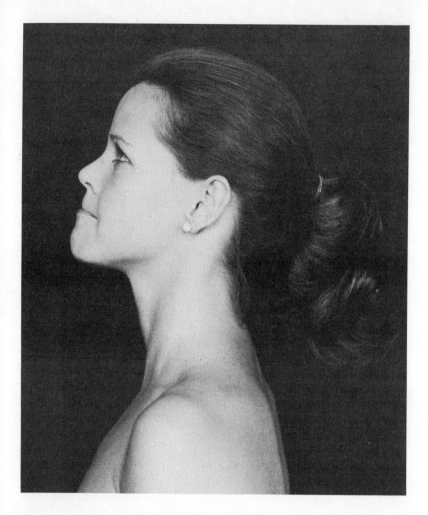

hard as possible. Your lower lip should cover the upper lip. Try to stretch it to meet the base of the nose.

There should be a pulling tension in the muscles under the chin.

Pull as hard as possible so you feel the tug under the point of the chin.

Mentally count to fifteen or let fifteen seconds pass.

Relax your face; let all muscles relax.

Repeat three times.

Lifting and Toning Muscles of the Lower Face; Toning Muscles of the Neck; Keeping the Muscles Around the Ears Flexible

(Cream needed)

Use ample amounts of nourishing and lubricating cream. Cover the ear area completely.

You will be using both hands. This is a two-part exercise.

1. Place the first finger of the right hand, the index finger, in back of the right ear. The middle finger of the hand goes in front. Both fingers should be as close as possible to the ear. The palm of your hand will rest against your well-creamed face.

Place the fingers firmly on flesh and move the entire hand in a complete circle, moving the tissue beneath the fingers.

Press upward, backward, then down and around. The flesh should be loosened gently but firmly.

The fingers should not move, but the four fingers that are used should move the skin and muscle over the hard bone that is in back of the ear.

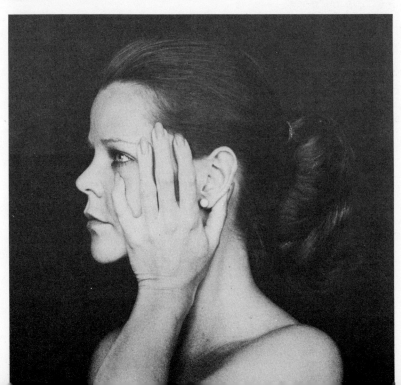

Repeat the circular massage five times.

You can use both the right and left hands, and tone the muscles on both sides of the face at the same time.

2. Place your hands with the fingers on either side of the ears, as in the first part of this exercise.

Push upward on the flesh around the right ear; at the same time, drag downward on the flesh around the left ear. The downward motion should pull until the fingers reach the base of the neck, the hollow under the earlobe directly in back of the jawbone.

Without lifting your fingers, reverse the direction of the hands, the left hand pushing upward to the top of the head and the right dragging down to the base of the neck.

Repeat the raising-lowering movement fourteen times (seven times for each ear in each direction).

Filling out the Neck; Aiding a Graceful Carriage of the Head

(Cream needed)

There are four parts to this exercise. Cream the jaw, neck, and shoulders carefully.

1. Bend the head backward as far as possible. Try to have it rest on the middle back.

Contract the muscles in the front of the neck, making them rigid, tensing the muscles of the neck.

Close the teeth and tense jaws until the cords on the neck stand out.

Open and close the mouth five times.

Keeping the teeth clenched, the neck muscles tense, and the cords on the neck taut, slowly raise the head to a vertical position.

While raising the head, keep the chin down, and push tension toward the back of the neck.

Repeat six times.

2. Position your head as in step 1, with your head back resting on the middle back, and teeth tightly clenched.

Turn your head so you are looking directly over your right shoulder.

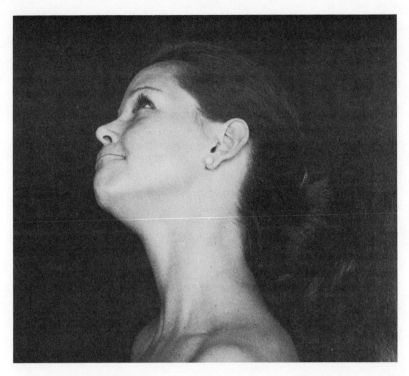

Count to four.

Keeping your head turned to the right, use the fingers of your left hand to gently rub and massage the left side of your neck using a rotary motion — upward and outward.

Reverse position of head, keeping it back; it should be turned to the left as far as possible.

Count to four.

With your right hand, massage the right side of your neck as described above.

Repeat the movement; six times left, six times right, massaging the neck each time.

Note: Keep teeth tightly clenched and muscles taut.

3. Position your head and tense the muscles as in step 1.

With the tips of your fingers, gently slap the skin on the sides of the neck.

Keep the teeth closed and neck tense while stimulating the neck with gentle slaps.

Note: The blood supply which nourishes the skin tissue is stimulated by the massage and tiny slaps.

4. Keep the head erect; relax face.

Place the palm of your left hand flat against the back of the neck at the hairline.

Place your right hand directly over the left. Keep both hands flat.

Press the hands forward tightly against the neck, and push backward against the resisting hands with all the strength of the neck and shoulders.

Hold this position during the count of five.

Relax, lower hands.

Repeat five times.

Lifting Sagging or Dips at the Sides of the Chin

(Cream needed)

The laxity of the muscles on the side of the chin causes the sagging; this movement exercises those muscles. The muscles at the sides of the face will become tense during the exercise, but ignore these side muscles.

Hold the chin firmly but do not press hard enough to bruise or mark the skin. Two hands are used, one hand on top of the other.

Open jaws and mouth.

Grasp chin firmly with one or both hands. Hold jaw open with hands.

Close jaw very slowly while strongly resisting the closing with the hand-held chin. Keep chin down and jaws out and open, resisting urge to close mouth. Concentrate on sides of chin.

Count to 25 slowly while resisting.

Relax.

Repeat three times.

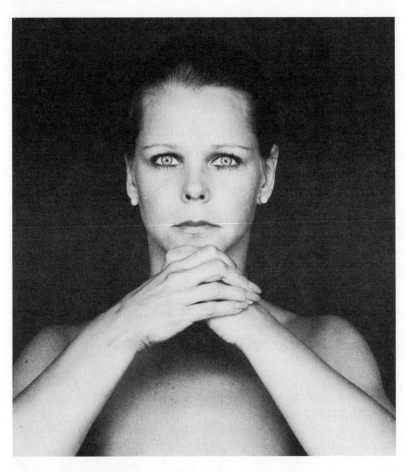

Firming Contour of Under-Chin and Front of Throat
(No cream needed)

This exercise may be skipped unless the chin is very heavy and the front of the throat is very sunken. Several other exercises can be used for most contouring and throat-front firming. See pages 58–64.

Place both hands on the forehead, fingers overlapping, palms down. Exert strong pressure on the forehead just above the brows. (The eyes may be covered by the position of the hands.)

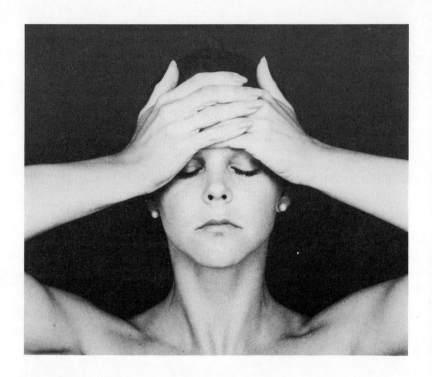

Raise arms to keep elbows level with the pressing hands.

Push head forward and downward. Resist this strongly with both hands and both arms. Do not drop elbows.

Continue trying to force the head down until you feel the muscles under the chin and on the throat tensing.

The head can be pushed downward against resistance until the chin almost touches the chest.

Push and resist, counting 15 and 25.

Relax. Allow hands and arms to drop.

Repeat exercise one to three times.

Note: Resisting the forward push of the head with your arms strongly tenses the muscles under the chin and in the front of the neck.

Firming under the Chin; Firming the Jaw and Lower- and Under-Cheek; Erasing Lines on the Sides of the Face; Erasing Horizontal Wrinkles on Neck

(Cream needed)

Sudden or jerky movements of the head when you are doing any exercise, and especially a neck exercise, can cause temporary dizziness and nausea. If *any* discomfort occurs, immediately abandon the exercise and check with your physician.

All neck exercises must be done slowly; this is also true of face-firming exercises. Ideally, you must pull very deeply on the muscles; otherwise exercising will only stretch the skin.

Stretch the neck upward; the chin should be thrust more upward than outward.

Turn your head to the left as far as possible. You should be able to look over your left shoulder.

The muscles of the neck should be taut and pulled hard as you turn. Draw your lower lip over the upper lip as you turn your head. This will increase pull on your neck muscles.

Hold neck tense, turned to left as far as possible, for the count of 15 to 25.

Concentrate on the muscles of the neck and the underside of the face as you hold the position. If you have difficulty exerting a strong and stretching pull on the muscles of the chin and neck, clasp your hands behind your neck and bring your elbows as close together in front as possible. This will pull the front chest and neck muscles downward, providing the resistance to your upward-thrust chin.

Keeping tension on the neck and chin, slowly return your head from the left-looking position to a forward position.

Relax.

Repeat movement five times to the left, and five times to the right.

Note: The hard pull on the neck-chin muscles must be exerted whenever the neck is turning as well as during the counts. The results depend on sufficient stretching and working of the neck and chin muscles.

Rounding a Thin Neck and Bony Shoulders
(Cream needed)

Cream the neck and upper shoulders. Use plenty of nourishing cream for this two-part exercise. The motions of this exercise should be gentle and soothing. Be careful not to pull the skin.

After exercising, blot and wipe away the skin cream. Follow with a freshening skin tonic such as witch hazel. Allow the tonic to remain on your skin for ten minutes. Then stimulate your neck, shoulders and chest with splashes of cold water. This will invigorate your skin and improve blood circulation.

This is a two-part exercise that is designed to free the muscles of the sides of the neck. You should feel a strong pull as you bend your head and bring it forward and backward.

1. Bend the head to the right.

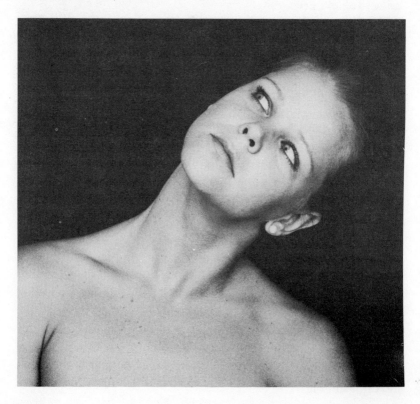

Keep the head bent over the right shoulder; your right ear should touch your right shoulder. Swing your head forward and backward.

Repeat, seven times forward and seven times backward.

Straighten your head.

Bend head to the left, and repeat the same action over the left shoulder.

Note: It is impossible to round and plump your neck if you carry your head and shoulders at a forward angle. If you have "neck hollows," try to relax, move more slowly, and gain weight if your shoulders and body are too thin.

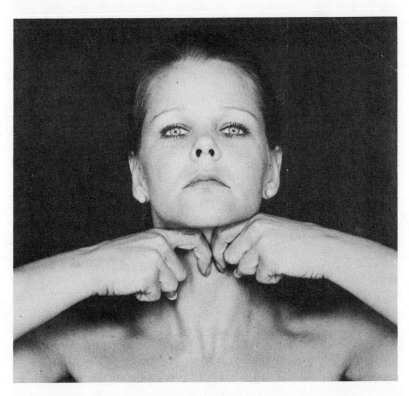

2. Bend your fingers; you will be using the area of the outside of the first and second joints, the knuckles.

Place the knuckles of both hands under your chin.

Bring them soothingly across the creamed under-chin and jawbone. Move from the middle of the neck, just under the chin, outward to follow the jawbone to under the ear. You should not pull the skin, but use a firm medium pressure up from the neck to the chin.

Repeat ten times.

You now have a selection of dozens of exercises at your disposal. Many of these can be done several times a day. The Basic Program, augmented by these additional exercises, will ensure dramatic results in a short time.

Many of my students plan their exercise program to look their best for some special occasion — such as a holiday or wedding — but you can start at any time, and something wonderful will happen!

PART FOUR

Do's and Don'ts—
Hints and Habits

I've received thousands of letters with questions and requests for advice. In this section I've tried to answer the most frequently asked questions and to organize and simplify the answers into hints and special tips. Presented in this way, they are so easy to remember that you can keep this knowledge with you at all times.

This section of the book provides tips, ideas, "secrets" that can be used in addition to exercises. All of these ideas can be used separately or in combination with the basic program or the combined basic and special program.

The first "secret" is sort of a special bonus. It is an exciting and amazing way to make your skin youthful and taut. If you want to look like a movie star, try it — it is the same technique some movie stars use.

Ice Water Skin Secrets

Sophia Loren and Paul Newman are two of the stars who use this ice water pack method to stimulate circulation in the skin and help promote tight pores, a firm tone, and a youthful dewy glow. It is the "stars' secret" for staying young.

1. Clean your face carefully; use a shower cap, or pin the hair back.

2. Fill the bathroom sink with two quarts of cold water. If the tap water is not cold, use water that has been kept in the refrigerator.

3. Place two full trays of ice cubes in a large piece of cheesecloth or a large handkerchief, and tie the ends so that the ice cubes will stay inside the cloth.

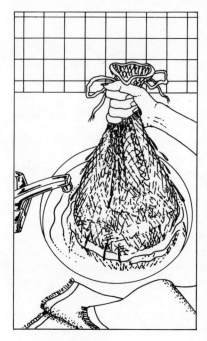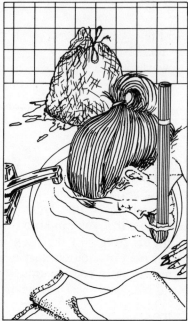

4. Place the bag of ice cubes into the cold water in the sink basin. *Never* put loose cubes into the water.

5. Dip your face into the icy water. Keep your face underwater for a minimum of 20 seconds in the beginning. (Later, see if you can keep your face underwater for 30 seconds, and later even more.) A small skin diver's snorkle can be used to keep your face underwater for longer than you can hold your breath. Paul Newman uses a snorkle.

6. Let your skin guide you. If a tingling sensation becomes uncomfortable, lift your head from the water.

7. When you remove your face from the water, lightly pat the skin dry. Use a very soft towel; do not rub.

8. Spray your face with mineral water.

9. Apply a light moisturizer to the entire face.

All About Bathing

All life comes from the sea. Seaside vacations are often suggested for relaxation, and people of all ages enjoy frolicking in the surf. However, those who are especially sensitive to cold and to the sun find such vacations unpleasant.

Thanks to modern science, we can now enjoy the benefits of salt water bathing in our own homes.

Jacuzzi baths, or similar baths that use bubbling water or jet sprays of various forces and temperatures, are a marvel of modern health equipment.

The reason that water therapy is effective is probably the fact that two-thirds of the body is liquid, and the body fluids themselves are similar in salt composition to the sea water. The mineral-rich water of the ocean can provide you with the natural massaging action of the waves. If you relax just at the water's edge and allow the waves to wash against your body, you'll be relaxed, refreshed, and invigorated by the sea water massage.

Stress, Worry, and Fear

Stress is your skin's worst enemy. Stress is the spring or mechanism that gets you going, but too much stress can cause problems—acne, wrinkles, or even a heart attack! There can be no beauty or real health when fear and worry take charge of your life. Stress and worry etch lines on the face and cause premature aging of the face and body.

What you think and feel, you become. Try to discard from your mind the thought of fear, worry, and uncertainty. They can only bring failure and disaster to your life. You cannot get the most out of life until you have learned to conquer fear, worry, and great amounts of stress.

Instead of running away from your problems, meet them with a sane, sensible solution. Remember, good thoughts are an armor against problems. Think yourself young and beautiful, even think of yourself as a person with a great figure, and that is who you will become.

Keep your mind so filled with love and beauty and positive thoughts that worry cannot enter.

Bad Habits for Firm Faces: Don'ts

1. Don't rest your face against your hand. The lines that develop will become permanent.

2. Don't slouch. Sit up straight; good posture is very important for keeping a youthful-looking neck.

3. Don't chew your food on only one side of your mouth. See your dentist to correct teeth problems. Chewing on one side develops the muscles on that side.

4. Don't wrinkle your nose when you smile or laugh. The correct way of laughing or smiling is stretching the mouth towards lobes of the ears.

5. Don't laugh moving the skin towards your temples. Crinkling your temples will cause lines to form around your eyes.

6. Don't squint when you laugh or smile. Squinting causes lines to form around your eyes.

7. Don't flash or move your eyebrows up when talking or gesturing. Keeping your forehead and face straight, smooth, and relaxed will keep your skin smooth.

8. Don't look into the bright sunlight without a good pair of sunglasses. Squinting from bright sunlight causes a network of lines around your eyes. The squint lines will become deeper and deeper, becoming a permanent part of your face.

9. Don't use a medium or large pillow. A baby pillow is best, or use a U-shaped neck pillow. During the night your face presses down deep into a large pillow. When you wake up in the morning, the skin has been pressed and folded; it takes an hour or so before these wrinkles finally fade away. After a few years, the lines will become permanent. Any pillow you use should be made of pure soft goose down.

10. Don't go out in cold weather without wearing gloves. To prevent wrinkles and age spots on the hands, you must protect the hands from the ravages of weather and of working and playing outdoors. Use rubber gloves also for washing dishes and cleaning, and use gloves for gardening or any heavy work, especially if you are using cleaners or solvents. (A bonus will be nice nails.)

Good Habits for Firm Faces: Do's

1. Do drink at least six glasses of water each day.

2. Do spray your skin with mineral water before applying any cream or makeup, and several times during each day.

3. Do eat good nutritious foods. Be sure you include fresh fruit and vegetables in your daily diet.

4. Do get at least seven hours of sleep every night.

5. Do sleep on a flat pillow, not a large soft pillow.

6. Do exercise your body as well as your facial muscles every day.

7. Do try to keep a happy, positive attitude about life.

8. Do clean your skin carefully; rid the surface of dead cells and stale creams and makeup.

9. Do protect your skin from sudden changes in temperature.

10. Do exercise your facial muscles for fifteen minutes each day.

Diet and Skin

Exercise alone cannot produce results unless you combine it with an entire new approach to beauty. That may include a change in diet, physical activity, and the way you breathe.

Diet does not necessarily mean that you should lose weight. Lines sometimes appear after a dramatic weight loss, and many people should actually gain weight. You should gain muscle, not fat weight. Filling out your facial muscles through a planned program of development can add inches and pounds to your neck, cheeks, and shoulders. The firm musculature of youth not only is desirable but ensures the proper blood supply with beauty-giving nutrients to your skin. One of the best basic diet programs is described in a free booklet published by the U.S. Government. It's called "The Prudent Diet"* and you can have it mailed to you by writing to the Bureau of Nutrition, Department of Health, Health Services Administration, New York, N.Y. 10013. Most nutritious

---

The Prudent Diet helps control weight and maintain it.

foods are the purest, with the most natural nutrients. Meat, fish, chicken,* fresh vegetables, and fruit should all be mainstays of your daily diet.

How active are you? The flexibility and grace of a youthful body that will complement your youthful face requires a program of body exercises and an active life style.

Breathing is vital to life: learn or relearn that breathing deeply and enjoying activity in the out-of-doors are part of an entire health and facial restructuring.

Soap

You cannot look your best unless your face is absolutely clean. I recommend washing with soap and water. Almost everyone should use soap for a thorough cleaning, but be careful: you must use the right soap for your skin. If you have dry or oily skin or a problem complexion, be sure the soap you use is aimed at helping to correct the condition. Soap formulas vary greatly.

Soaps such as Dove contain ingredients that are very mild and are usually compatible with even the most sensitive skin. These are the best types of soaps to use for a normal to dry skin.

An oily skin should be cleaned with a less fatty soap. Oatmeal soap and some of the sea soaps that contain small particles to act as gentle abrasives are wonderful for cleansing the outer surfaces of the skin and ridding the skin of oily plugs. Brasovil is the brand name of this kind of soap.

Cleansing Your Face Without Soap

Some people have skin that cannot tolerate soap. These people — everyone else, for that matter — can use this wonder cleansing oil. It's an excellent cleanser, better than any of the commercial

---

*A vegetarian should read the book, *Diet for a Small Planet*, by Frances Moore Lappe. It is a guide to high-protein meatless cooking.

cleansing creams or lotions sold. You can make it yourself at home. Here is the recipe (use only cold pressed oils):

1 ounce sunflower oil
1 ounce avocado oil
2 ounces sesame oil

Combine these three oils in a small jar that has a tight lid on top. Shake gently to mix.

This liquid cleanser can be stored without refrigeration. It is excellent for removing eye makeup because it is gentle to the most delicate skin.

When removing the wonder cleansing oil from your skin, never, *never* use tissue. Tissues are made from wood pulp and even the finest tissues can leave microscopic splinters on the skin. Instead, wipe the face gently with disposable cotton balls or swatches of absorbent cotton.

Clean Your Face and Face the World

At least once a day use soap and water to clean your face completely. You may use the wonder cleansing oil in the morning if you have extremely dry skin, but nothing takes the place of soap for spic and span cleaning. Do not use a cleansing cream at night; it doesn't clean as easily and thoroughly as soap. At night, soap is a must! Here is the best way to really cleanse your face.

1. Fill the sink or a basin with warm water.

2. Wet face.

3. Dip the soap in the water. Lather soap in your hands.

4. Apply the soapy lather to your face in an upward motion. Move the lather up and away from the face. Always wash upward. I use a *natural boar-bristle complexion brush;* I have found it does wonders in ridding the face of grime. *Never* use a *nylon* complexion brush or a washing sponge. If you want to use a washcloth, use it, but use it only once. Bacteria collect on a wet washcloth and can cause trouble.

5. Rinse your face at least 40 times with fresh water, by splashing water on your face. A good technique is to splash-press the rinse water to your face. Use clean running water, not too hot, just tepid.

6. Pat your skin dry with a soft clean towel. Be careful not to mash your nose or drag your skin in any way.

7. Spray the face with mineral water from an atomizer.

8. Apply a rich moisturizer on top of the wet sprayed skin. Never put any moisturizer or cream on a dry face. Don't dip your fingers into the jar; use a clean spatula or spoon. This method will keep the cream free of contamination.

9. At night apply a good, rich protein night cream.

Beware of the Sun

1. Avoid sunbathing between 11:00 A.M. and 3:00 P.M. This is when the sun is at its highest and the rays are most intense. If you want to sunbathe, it is much safer in the morning or late afternoon.

2. Never, never use a sun reflector.

3. Do not go in the sun immediately after a meal.

4. Always use a 5% PABA* cream, lotion, or gel on the body and a sun block on your face. Do not use anything but a 5% PABA and a sun block. Spray your face and body with mineral water before and after applying the PABA.

5. Spray your body with a mineral water spray as often as possible when you are in the sun. This spraying will help the skin to keep its moisture level.

6. Avoid sunbathing and bright sunlight when you are taking any medication or drugs. The sun may cause a reaction with the drugs in your body. Check with your doctor.

7. Windy days can be harmful to your skin; the wind can hasten sunburn. The wind, even a cool wind, dries out the oil and moisture of your skin, leaving it dry and unprotected.

*PABA stands for *paraminobenzoic acid.*

Beauty Sleep

The phrase "beauty sleep" is very apt. The right amount of sleep is important to your appearance. Try to get an average of eight hours a night, or at least seven hours, if that seems all that is possible. You cannot look fresh and rested with less. Sleep is necessary for replenishing your energy and it is relaxation that is vital for daytime energy and stamina. Sleep is rejuvenating for the face and body; it dissipates tension and is a respite from strain on the glands and nervous system. Lack of sleep causes poor muscle tone and accentuates wrinkles. Sleep only on a baby pillow, neck rest, or beauty pillow.

Water, Water, Water

Water is the ultimate moisturizer for your skin. It is vital for proper skin care; it is the single most important element for avoiding or postponing wrinkles. You need water both inside and outside. Drinking water is one of the best things you can do for your skin. I drink a minimum of seven glasses of water a day. I think it is a great cleanser, and it also helps to improve the complexion.

Humidifiers

Unfortunately, most apartments and houses need to be heated in the wintertime. The heat evaporates the moisture in the air, so that even plants beg for water. Invest in a room or home humidifier, which will put additional water into the air. Your entire family will be healthier too. Very dry air dries out the membranes of the nose and throat and can create an environment that invites infection. A humidifier or room moisturizer will also help you prevent dehydrated skin.

If you don't want to invest in a humidifier, place a pan of water on the top of the radiator or near the heat source. It works almost as well as a commercial humidifier.

Dehydrated Skin

Dehydrated skin can be oily skin. The skin has enough oil but not enough moisture, that is, water. Dehydrated skin is usually caused by overexposure to the sun, or hot or windy climates. It can often result from indoor heating systems that rob the air of all its moisture and encourage evaporation of the moisture in the skin.

Oily Skin

Oily skin may have a tendency to blemish, but it has the virtue of keeping wrinkles away for a long time. Oily skin is often accompanied by enlarged pores. When the skin is not correctly cleaned, the pores become clogged. The air causes the oil to discolor and the grease and dirt become blackheads.

The use of a good exfoliation cream is a must to prevent the buildup of clogging oil. There are many good exfoliation creams on the market.

Another way to control an oily skin is from within, by changing your eating habits: don't eat fatty foods, overprocessed foods, candy, cake, pie, sweets, or fried foods. Be sure to include raw salads with leafy greens in them and to drink fruit and vegetable juices.

Dry Skin

Dry skin does not have enough water and protective oil. Dry skin can usually be traced to improper care. Most people do not know how to use a good night cream, so the creams, no matter how expensive, do not work.

To get the best out of your cream, spray the face with mineral water before applying the cream. After the face has been moisturized, apply a protein cream.

Hints

1. Don't ever put a moisturizer or a cream on a dry, unsprayed skin.

2. Don't grimace; eventually grimacing will put wrinkles and creases in your face.

3. Never use facial tissues on your skin. Tissues contain wood pulp, which can irritate your skin.

4. Hormones of any kind, as well as birth control pills, can cause trouble for your skin.

5. Never go outdoors without covering your skin. There is a myth that your skin must breathe; it is only a myth. A face without protection allows the environment pollutants to attack your skin.

6. Never put perfume directly on your skin.

7. Twenty minutes a day on the wonderful slant board will help improve muscle tone.

8. Exercise your complete body for beautiful facial skin. To my surprise I have found that exercising the body improves the entire complexion.

9. When you are on a diet, never lose more than 2 pounds a week; a drastic weight loss can cause you to lose muscle tone.

10. Don't take any drugs without the advice of your doctor.

11. Think young and beautiful and you will become young and beautiful.

12. Never slouch in your chair. Your posture when sitting, standing, and walking will affect your facial skin.

APPENDIX

Hollywood Instant Face Lift

The only way to really reverse the effects of time is through consistent exercise. But, for a very special occasion, when you really want to look your best instantly, there is a way you can look up to twenty years younger. *Caution:* Reserve this trick for just once in a great while. It is great for a party, an interview, or having your picture taken; it isn't for everyday.

You'll need some special materials: Micropore surgical tape is an almost transparent tape that is used in operations; it is so strong and so durable that it can be used by a doctor directly over a wound. The tape is made by the 3M Company of Minneapolis. This tape comes in many widths but you will need a roll of the ¾-inch width. Check several drugstores and pharmacies; you will probably be able to buy it locally. If it is not available, or if you prefer, you can also use Band-Aid Clear Tape, made by Johnson & Johnson. This also comes in several widths, but again, you'll need the ¾-inch width. (The second method described below uses only this Band-Aid tape.)

For the second method you will also need a large needle with a large eye, or a small hole punch; and about 24 inches of strong twine or plastic line such as fishing line.

There are two methods of using the tapes. Either method works; however, some people prefer to use the string-tie method for longer periods of time, or for their face, and the tape-only method for their neck.

Before beginning you'll have to make some plans. It is important to select a hair style that will cover the tapes when they are positioned on the sides of your face and neck. You cannot wear your hair back, off the face and neck, or in a very smooth style.

If your hair is at least chin length, hiding the face lift will be easiest.

Here is how you can "roll back the years" with the use of these tapes.

1. Wash and dry your face thoroughly. Do not use cream; use soap and water, rinse, and pat dry. With a ball of cotton, cleanse the sides of your face with alcohol to be sure the face is perfectly clean — without a trace of oil, even the natural oil from the skin — and very dry.

2. Cut the tapes into 2-inch-long pieces. Lay several cut tapes, gum-side up, in front of you. Seat yourself before a mirror.

Method 1

1. Place the flat of your index finger at the outside end of your eye. Now push and slide your finger toward the sideburn — head toward the little button of cartilege at the point in the middle of the ear. Force the skin before your pushing finger, to the sideburn area. Attach the tape firmly to the fold of skin that is bunched in front of the ear. Press firmly. Repeat the procedure on the other side of the face.

2. Run your finger from the side of your mouth to under your earlobe, pushing and sliding the skin in the same way you did in the outer eye area. Tape the excess skin firmly to hold it back from the center face.

Note: Be sure to use the same tension on both sides of the face. Don't make the skin unnaturally tight. Remember you will have to move, talk, and perhaps eat or drink with the lift in place.

3. Repeat the same procedure on the other side of your face.

4. Starting at the center of the throat, just under the chin, run your finger along the jawline and back toward the ear, and under the earlobe. Tape the excess skin on the side of the back of the neck. Repeat on the other side of the throat, and tape securely.

Using this tape method you can temporarily trim sagging skin from your chin and jaw, fill out hollows and lines, and erase the bags under the eyes.

Method 2

In this method, the only tape that you should use is Band-Aid Clear Tape from Johnson & Johnson.

1. Use the ¾-inch width tape, and cut several pieces 2½-inches long. Fold the end of each piece of tape back about ¼-inch, just enough to provide a nonsticky double-tape surface. Allow about 2-inches of the tape to remain sticky. Using a large needle or a hole punch, make a small hole in the center of the folded section of the tape. Tie a strong, thin string or a plastic line about 12 inches long to the tape. You should have two or more folded pieces of tape with strings attached before going to the next step.

2. Using the same techniques as in Method 1, slide and push your loose skin from the center of your face to just in front of the ear. Apply the tape with the string hanging down.

3. Repeat so you have both sides taped and a length of string hanging on each side of the face.

4. Tie the string together; tie snugly, but not too tightly, on the top of the head.

5. Hide the string under your hair; carefully arrange the hair over the "lift."

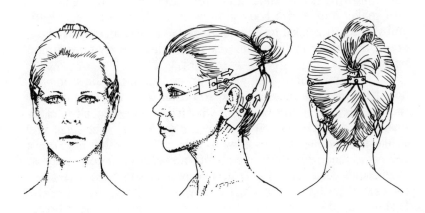

Note: Heavy or opaque makeup can be used over the tapes for extra camouflage. This might be useful especially for the sides of the face, near the ears.

The lifts should hold for many hours.

Remove the tape lifts carefully. When it comes time to take them off, be very gentle. Hold the skin with the fingers of one hand as you gently pull the sticking tape with the other.

After the tape has been removed, clean any gum or sticky residue from the skin with alcohol; then wash the face carefully, spray with water, and apply a moisturizer. Be very generous in applying the moisturizer to the part of the skin that has been moved by the tapes or was under the tape.

These temporary lifts are not good for your skin. Do not use them often. Save this trick for a very special occasion.

Total Skin Care
(The Dry-Brush Bath for a Soft Skin and a Healthy Glowing Face and Body)

The following is a method of cleaning and massaging the skin. It will make your entire body glow with newly-stimulated health and vitality. It is good for your skin and as an extra bonus it invigorates the entire body and leaves you feeling newly-minted and polished.

Just as pollution, dust, grease, grime, and dirt collect on windowsills, inside clothes cabinets, and even seep into locked cases, they collect on our own protective covering—our skin. This unwanted residue, combined with our own dead skin cells, prevents the natural healthy glow of the skin from showing. (Skin cells grow, mature, and die in about four weeks—callouses are an example of dead cells that collect to protect stress areas.) Instead the skin is dull and sallow with scaly peeling areas and blotches. Dirt and dead cells are unhealthy, too. They are excellent breeding grounds for bacteria. A dry-brush bath rids the skin of all this unneeded and unwanted material.

The only equipment needed is a natural-bristle brush or a scrubber made of a natural material. The best of the natural fibers is goat hair, next best is a boar bristle, but be sure it is soft enough to feel comfortable. However, don't use a nylon or synthetic-fiber brush. They can be harmful to the skin. Even some soft sponge-like synthetics that are well advertised should not be used. They have a tendency to scratch the skin. Just be sure the scrubber or brush you use is from a natural source.

To keep your natural-bristle brush clean and sweet smelling, be sure it is carefully rinsed after every use in very hot water. Don't just swish the bristles through the water, be sure that any dead skin or dirt that might be lodged between the bristles is washed away and the base of the brush is free of any foreign particles. Every few days, or at least once a week, you should soap and rinse the brush and let it dry completely in a warm place that has a good circulation of fresh air. Some people like to keep two brushes so that one is ready to use at all times.

You might want to start with a fast 5-minute dry bath. And you should try this technique twice a day. The dry bath should usually take about 15 minutes. Don't overdo, especially in the beginning. A 10-minute dry bath is better than a 15-minute bath that leaves you raw and feeling scratched. Your own sensitivity will let you know exactly when you've had enough.

The best time for a dry bath is before your daily or twice-daily shower. Or, if you don't bathe or shower after the dry bath, you can sponge your body lightly with water (cool, tepid, or warm — whatever your preference may be) to take away any old skin cells and other debris that might be on your newly cleaned and glowing skin. No matter when it is most convenient for you, remember, don't overdo.

Many people find a dry-brush bath is a wonderful wakeup for their entire body in the morning, and a relaxing end to a busy day. When you brush-massage your body and limbs just before going to bed you'll probably wake up feeling well-rested and smooth.

Here are directions for a dry bath:

1. Start at your toes and feet, use circular overlapping strokes.
2. Rub and brush the toes, soles of your feet and arches, work toward the heel and be very gentle in rubbing and massaging the ankles.

3. Work upward, both front and back of the leg. The legs can be brushed either in a sitting position or while standing. Many people find it easy to rest one leg on the edge of the bathtub.
4. Work over the knees and be sure that the outer thighs are well-brushed. Don't forget the back of the legs and the rough skin that may be on your upper thigh.
5. Do not brush your sex organs or delicate parts of the body, but do not forget the buttocks and the hips.
6. Work gently up the body and over the breasts. Support your breast with one hand as you very gently dry brush the skin with your other hand.
7. The back and shoulders can be reached when you attach a hand strap to your brush. The motion of the rubbbing is as good for your upper arms as it is for your skin — it helps to firm the muscles of the upper arm.
8. Don't forget the joint of the armpit. Be very careful under the arm, but you can be quite firm on the outer section of arm and the shoulders.
9. Brush the back of your neck in a circular motion; working up from the shoulders to the hairline. Be gentle as you brush the throat and use only an upward motion, up under the chin and to the earlobes.
10. Work the brush upward on your face; go up the sides and across the cheeks. Do not try to go near the eyes, but if you have heavy brows brush them gently. Be very careful not to mash your nose, or pull or drag any of the skin on your throat or face.
11. Carefully brush the hairline to be sure you get rid of any dry skin that might have accumulated.

Now your skin is clean and stimulated. A few minutes under the running water of the shower will wash away all loosened and dead skin and any foreign matter. No soap is needed nor should it be used.

After drying yourself lightly, spray your face and body with mineral water from a small spray bottle. Then over the mineral water apply a light cover of oil such as cold, pressed avocado oil. You'll notice how quickly it seems to combine with your skin and how delicate and soft your skin feels. And, best of all, you've just given yourself a beauty-health treat that will

- Keep your pores clean and reduce blemishes and blackheads.
- Free your skin of dead cells so that it is younger looking and clearer, and has fewer discolorations.
- Encourage an even distribution of body fat; the brushing helps to rid the body of lumps and fat deposits on your upper thighs and upper arms, or on the buttocks or across the stomach or around the waist.
- Stimulate the nerve endings on the skin surface; this stimulation is good for the entire nervous system.
- Excite the tiny blood vessels and so help to encourage a good blood supply to the skin surface and circulation in the entire body.

The Russians have used this method of skin care for centuries and they often brush their limbs and body with oak leaves and branches instead of a natural bristle brush. Many Scandinavians use variations of a dry-brush bath in their saunas. It is an excellent skin treatment for winter-chapped or summer's sun-peeling skin; it is perfect for all-year, all-body beauty.

Resource List

Cream and Moisturizer, Soap, Protein Cream* Catalog

Jon Suarse Inc.
P.O. Box 634
F.D.R. Station
New York, New York 10022

How to Make Juice Mask

J. E. Kiement
Acme Juicer Co.
1031 Main Avenue
Clifton, New Jersey 07011

Vitamin and Mineral Catalogs

L & H
1062 Lexington Avenue
New York, New York 10021

Water

Mountain Valley Water
150 Central Avenue
Hot Springs, Arkansas 71901
Toll-free :(800)643-1150

Take a picture of your face when starting my exercises, and
again after six months. For any information about my Natural
Skin Care Course, write to:
M. J. Saffon
P.O. Box 23
Lenox Hill Station
New York, New York 10021

*Protein cream is any cream that has collagen protein in it.

Index

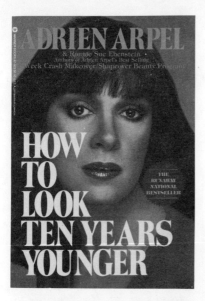

If you found THE 15-MINUTE-A-DAY NATURAL FACELIFT useful, you will find Adrien Arpel's

HOW TO LOOK TEN YEARS YOUNGER

a must also. Ms. Arpel, president of her own multi-million-dollar cosmetics company, tells you:

- How to give yourself a 10-years-younger image in just one day via her 5-step repackaging system
- How to do the Body Lift—the 10-minutes-a-day, 10-years-off body tune-up that lifts and firms every part of your anatomy
- How to follow the 24-Hour Emergency! Diet—the doctor's healthy way to lose 2 or more pounds in just one day
- How to dress to hide body flaws: The Clothes Camouflage Workshop
- How make-up can shape down a full face . . . hide first lines
- How to grow a lush, young-looking head of hair: the vitamins, minerals and foods that promote luxuriant hair
- How to enter the hair color Time Machine (and exit looking 10 years younger, 10 times more fantastic)
- How to win the Big Six skin battles and be practically wrinkle-free after age 25

A large-format quality paperback

$7.95 (Canada, $8.95)
L97823-X (U.S.A.)
L97846-9 (Canada)

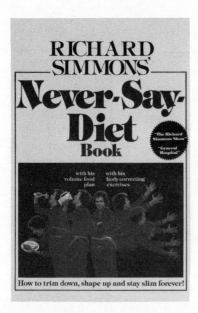